Notes on Paediatrics

Neurology

Alex Habel MBChB, FRCP, MRCPCH
Paediatrician, West Middlesex University Hospital;
Consultant Paediatrician, Great Ormond Street Children's Hospital,
London

Rod Scott MBChB, MRCP
Clinical Research Fellow, Institute of Child Health, London

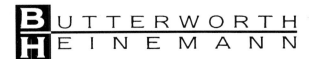

OXFORD   BOSTON   JOHANNESBURG   MELBOURNE   NEW DELHI   SINGAPORE

Butterworth-Heinemann
Linacre House, Jordan Hill, Oxford OX2 8DP
225 Wildwood Avenue, Woburn, MA 01801-2041
A division of Reed Educational and Professional Publishing Ltd

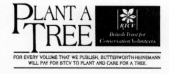 A member of the Reed Elsevier plc group

First published 1998

British Library Cataloguing in Publication Data
A catalogue record for this book is available from the British Library

Library of Congress Cataloguing in Publication Data
A catalogue record for this book is available from The Library of Congress

ISBN 0 7506 2445 0

27/8/98
M

Composition by Scribe Design, Gillingham, Kent
Printed and bound by MPG Books Ltd, Bodmin, Cornwall

PLANT A
TREE

British Trust for
Conservation Volunteers

FOR EVERY VOLUME THAT WE PUBLISH, BUTTERWORTH-HEINEMANN
WILL PAY FOR BTCV TO PLANT AND CARE FOR A TREE.

Contents

Introduction to the series

Originally, *Synopsis of Paediatrics* was written with an overriding awareness of the need for a carefully focused textbook for practical work on the wards and in preparing for examinations using the problem-orientated approach. This series is a response to requests from students and postgraduates for easily affordable, updated versions of the most used sections. Thus the first section of each volume is an addition to the original text, containing embryology, recent developments in pathophysiology and disease management issues. Some sections in the respiratory disease volume have been completely rewritten.

As with the complete volume of *Synopsis of Paediatrics*, we have selected topics for their relevance to clinical practice. Doctors in training have told us that references are rarely consulted in textbooks, despite the preconceptions of reviewers (usually senior paediatricians), especially as up to the minute CD ROM searches have become so accessible. They are therefore kept to a minimum. The aim of the synoptic approach is to provide a digest on which the users can develop their clinical approach. A problem-orientated and systems method has been synthesized. In this introduction we will also touch on concepts that underpin this way of practising medicine in the last decade of the twentieth century.

HOW TO MAKE BEST USE OF THE TEXT AND IMPROVE YOUR SKILLS

Deductive reasoning in establishing a diagnosis

The success of a problem-orientated approach lies in sifting the information obtained from the history and signs to identify a problem or problems, then generating a list of possible diagnoses. The construction of a hypothesis of most likely causation is tested by deductive reasoning, answers to questions and findings of a positive nature tending to confirm, negative responses to exclude. Clinically 80–85% of diagnoses can be reached in this way, aided by clinical examination, confirmation coming from investigation where appropriate. Investigations should be selected to help confirm or reject the veracity of the hypotheses. When non-contributory or contradictory, review the history and findings and consider what further causes are possible. The alternative blunderbuss approach is slow, cumbersome and costly in time and resources.

Evidence based medicine (EBM)

'EBM is the conscientious, explicit and judicious use of best current evidence in making decisions about the care of individual patients' (British Medical Journal, 1996). Although this approach is traditionally held to be the scientific basis of our system of medical practice a more critical appraisal of our use of examination, investigation and therapies has shown how shallow is that reality. We are increasingly asked to justify the clinical decisions we take, and this requires an awareness of published relevant clinical research experience. This is available on data bases such as the Cochrane Collaborative Project data base, and CD ROM and on-line computer searches of the journals. The aim is to integrate the best external evidence with individual clinical expertise. It also covers accuracy of diagnostic tests, prognosis, and physical therapies. We draw attention to this important development to orientate the student, be it at an undergraduate or postgraduate level, to the need to familiarize himself with this concept.

Reference

British Medical Journal (1996) Leader. Evidence based medicine: what it is and what it isn't. **312**, 71–72

Greenhalgh T (1997) How to read a paper. *The Basics of Evidence Based Medicine*. London: British Medical Journal

Abbreviations

Abbreviations have been kept to a minimum, and the following will be found in the text:

AD Autosomal dominant inheritance
AR Autosomal recessive inheritance
CT Computerized tomography
EEG Electroencephalograph
ESR Erythrocyte sedimentation rate
FBC Full blood count
LP Lumbar puncture
MRI Magnetic resonance imaging
US Ultrasound
WBC White blood count
XL Sex linked inheritance

EMBRYOLOGY

A basic knowledge of embryology is useful in understanding congenital abnormalities of the brain. There are three stages of morphogenesis.

1   Organogenesis: major brain development in first 4 weeks, completed by 9 weeks.
2   Cytogenesis: continuous multiplication and differentiation of cell lines. Pluripotential cell develops on the periventricular surface to form neuroblasts (→ neurons) and glioblasts (→ astrocytes, oligodendrocytes, microglia or ependymal cells).
3   Histogenesis is the process of cell migration, tissue formation and orientation of cells to each other and supporting tissues. Neuroblasts migrate along glial guides from the ventricular ependyma to the pial surface with the cells migrating last becoming the most superficial in the cortex, principally between 20 and 30 weeks' gestation (Figure 1).

Organogenesis will be described individually for clarity.

Organogenesis

Neurulation: the endodermal neural plate rolls up into the neural tube which closes up forming a fluid-filled cylinder.

Transverse segmentation: the cylinder initially divides into four segments. The prosencephalon and rhombencephalon divide again to leave six segments. From superior to inferior they are:

   i   Telencephalon: forms cerebral hemispheres.
  ii   Diencephalon: forms thalamus, hypothalamus and epithalamus.
 iii   Mesencephalon: forms midbrain.
 iv   Metencephalon: forms pons.

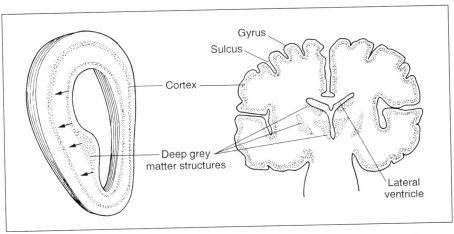

Figure 1   Migration of neuroblasts from periventricular matrix zone to cortex. Normal distribution of grey matter seen in right hand diagram

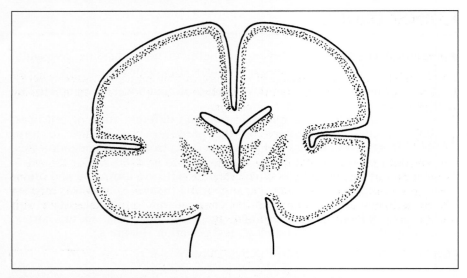

Figure 2   Lissencephaly. Failure in the development of gyri and sulci

    v Myelencephalon: forms medulla oblongata.
    vi Myelon: forms spinal cord.

Evagination of the neural tube walls to form the pineal, olfactory and optic bulbs, pituitary and cerebral hemispheres.

Flexion of neural tube forms adult configuration of brain structure.

Protusion of masses: differs from evagination in that the ventricular lumen is not included. Largest protuberance is the cerebellum.

Fissuring and sulcation of cerebrum and cerebellum.

Clinical relevance

1   Failure of neurulation: all neural tube defects including anencephaly, myelomeningocoele and sacral agenesis.
2   Failure of cerebral hemisphere separation: holoprosencephaly.
3   Disturbances of cerebellar morphogenesis: Dandy-Walker malformation, aplasia, Joubert syndrome.
4   Failure of normal histogenesis: neuronal migration defects, e.g. micrencephaly, megalencephaly, lissencephaly (Figure 2), pachygyria, polymicrogyria, grey matter heterotopia (Figures 3 and 4).

EPIDEMIOLOGY

Paroxysmal phenomena

Single most common neurological problem in childhood. Includes epilepsy, breath-holding attacks and faints. Prevalence was about 7% in a national British cohort, in which 4.1% had epilepsy.

Epilepsy

The overall prevalence of epilepsy is estimated to be 4–6/1000 for the whole population but this must be considered a conservative estimate. The prevalence in schoolchildren is of the order of 8/1000. Seizures occur in just over 1% of neonates. Seizures become less common with age, although there is another peak in prevalence in the elderly.

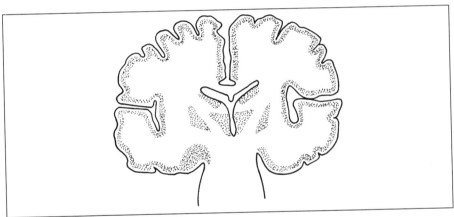

Figure 3 Focal area of mesial temporal cortical thickening

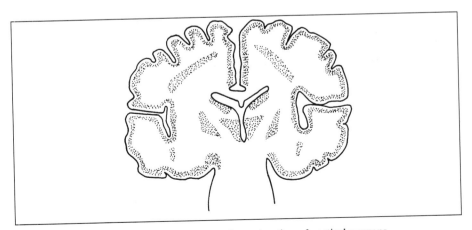

Figure 4 Band heterotopia. Failure of complete migration of cortical neurons

The incidence of epilepsy is 20–70/100 000 per year.

Status epilepticus occurs in 50 000–60 000 persons annually in the USA, the majority in children. Mortality is currently about 5% and is usually the result of an underlying condition.

Febrile convulsions

Fever is the commonest cause of seizure in childhood; 3–5% of the population will have at least one febrile convulsion and of those about 5% will have an episode of febrile status epilepticus. Compared with the normal population recent studies show a good outcome. There is much debate about whether febrile convulsions lead to an increased incidence of later afebrile seizures. Complex partial seizures caused by hippocampal (mesial temporal) sclerosis is relatively rare and 60% will have a past history of febrile convulsions. A national cohort study concluded that outcome is determined more by the underlying cause than the seizures themselves.

Febrile convulsions and anticonvulsant medication

Diazepam prophylaxis at the time of fever reduces the frequency of recurrence (12% vs 38%). However, diazepam treatment of seizures as they occurred has the same outcome as diazepam prophylaxis for epilepsy, intelligence, schooling and neurology. Therefore generally reserve prophylaxis for those with multiple, prolonged seizures or with a high risk of recurrence.

References

Knudsen F U, Paerregaard A, Andersen R, Andersen J (1996) Long term outcome of prophylaxis for febrile convulsions. *Archives of Disease in Childhood*, **74**, 13–18

Verity C M, Ross E M, Golding J (1993) Outcome of childhood status epilepticus and lengthy febrile convulsions: findings of national cohort study. *British Medical Journal*, **307**, 225–228

Neural tube defects

Neural tube defects continue to be much rarer than a decade ago due to effective antenatal ultrasound diagnostic services and subsequent termination of pregnancy. Healthy living campaigns for all women of child bearing age are targeting dietary folate (recommended 400 μg daily). In women on the anticonvulsants valproate and carbamazepine, this should be given preconception (5 mg daily) as the risk is 10 × greater.

Headache

Migraine is the most important cause in all age groups. The incidence of migraine increases with increasing age rising from 2.7% at age 7 to 6.4% of boys and 14.8% of girls at age 14 years. In one Maryland county in the USA 12% of adolescents missed a day of school in the preceding month because of headache; 13% of males and 20% of females will consult a doctor about headache and of these up to 8% will be referred to a neurologist. Headache is a major cause of morbidity especially in the adolescent age group.

NEUROCHEMISTRY

Neurotransmitters play a vital role in central nervous system functioning. They have a role in modulating both physiological and pathological mechanisms for motor, sensory and cognitive function. At least 70 neurotransmitters have been identified but the most studied ones in epilepsy are:

- Excitatory: glutamate, aspartate.
- Inhibitory: GABA, acetylcholine, dopa.

Neuronal death or damage is possibly due to excessive release of excitatory amino acids (EAA). Glutamate stimulates N-methyl-D-aspartate (NMDA) and non-NMDA receptors on the neuronal surface with the result that there is rapid calcium influx which promotes second and third messenger mechanisms with subsequent cell death.

Causes of excessive EAA release include:

- Trauma
- Seizures
- Hypoxia/ischaemia
- Intracranial infection.

Drugs that inhibit pathological release of excitatory amino acids may ultimately play a significant role in neuroprotection.

The role of neurotransmitters in epilepsy

Imbalance between EAA and inhibitory amino acids is the likely cause of seizure initiation, although this is probably a simplistic view.

This information is necessary for the understanding of the mechanisms of action of many of the anticonvulsants.

   i GABA agonists: vigabatrin, benzodiazepines (surprisingly, not gabapentine).

   ii Glutamate antagonists: remacemide, topiramate.

Another primary anti-seizure mechanism through blockage of voltage-sensitive sodium ion channels may account for the effects of carbemazepine, phenytoin, lamotrogine

Other roles for neurotransmitters

Neurotransmitters are also involved in cognition (and therefore imbalance may be responsible for some psychiatric conditions). Examples:

Serotonin (5-hydroxytriptamine; 5-HT) a neurotransmitter in brain, spinal cord and myenteric plexus. Drugs that alter the balance of 5-HT have profound effects on behaviour.

- Agonists: sumatriptan for migraine (blocks firing of the trigeminal ganglion which is now recognized as responsible for the painful headache, superseding the theory that constriction of dilated intracranial vessels is therapeutic).

Lithium in prophylaxis of manic depression (not in the paediatric age group).

- Antagonists: pizotifen in migraine prophylaxis. Ondansetron and granisetron for chemotherapy, postoperative and radiotherapy related emesis.
- 5-HT reuptake inhibitors: fluoxetine (Prozac) for depression, obsessive compulsive disorder, bulimia nervosa.
- 5-HT released: methylphenidate (Ritalin) in attention deficit hyperactivity disorder.

Selected effect of melatonin on sleep patterns in disabled children

Melatonin is the pineal hormone signalling sleep–wake cycles and has a rapid, transient mild sleep inducing effect. One study has shown significant improvement in improving the sleep pattern of multiply disabled children, using 2.5–10 mg melatonin.

Reference

Jan J E, Espezel H (1995) Melatonin treatment of chronic sleep disorders. *Journal of Developmental Medicine and Child Neurolology*, **37**, 279–280

GENETICS

Autosomal dominant: neurofibromatosis, tuberous sclerosis.
With genomic imprinting (the parental origin of the gene determines the phenotype): juvenile-onset Huntingdon's disease with seizures is likely to be inherited through the father.

Autosomal recessive: metabolic, e.g. phenylketonuria, Tay–Sachs disease.

X-linked: fragile X mental retardation.

Chromosomal: Down's syndrome.

Mitochondrial inheritance: maternally transmitted as all mitochondria are from the mother's ovum and males cannot transmit, e.g. Leigh's disease.
DNA studies: some epilepsies have shown linkage to candidate genes: the rare benign familial neonatal convulsions on chromosome 20, the relatively common juvenile myoclonic epilepsy to chromosome 6.
   Triplet repeats: excessive number of the same amino acid triplet code on the gene is responsible for fragile X (>50 repeats), and dystrophia myotonica.

Multifactorial: for siblings of someone with idiopathic epilepsy the general risk (4%) is 4 × general population (1%), rising to 8% if a parent is similarly affected, and up to 15% if a similar spike and wave EEG pattern is found. Risk to offspring is 3–4%.

SURGICAL TREATMENT OF EPILEPSY

Children appear to benefit more than adults. Suitable for generalized, but mainly used for partial seizures. Timing is a compromise between avoiding the disruption and psychological damage of continuing seizures against potential improvement in seizure frequency over time (Table 1).

Indications for surgery

Intractable disabling seizures for 2–4 years on optimal therapy. Non-progressive but without the likelihood of spontaneous recovery.

Aims

1   To remove where there is a primary focus or disconnect where removal is not possible.
2   Reduce the mass of neurons behaving abnormally.

Table 1   Types of surgery and their indication

Operation	Indication
Focal cortical resection	
Temporal	Partial seizures
Extratemporal	Focus of seizure localized clinically, and by EEG and imaging
Multiple subpial resections	Landau-Kleffner syndrome of speech and language regression + partial seizures
Corpus callosotomy	Intractable primary generalized tonic-clonic, atonic or myoclonic seizures
Hemispherectomy	Widespread origin of seizures in one damaged hemisphere

Results

When correctly selected preoperatively, 50–80% are significantly improved or seizure free.

NORMAL DEVELOPMENT

Skills are assessed in four areas of development:

- Gross motor activity.
- Fine motor and vision.
- Hearing and speech.
- Social behaviour and play.

1 Development normally advances synchronously between these areas.

Mental retardation often involves impaired or delayed fine motor and social behaviour, as well as language, while motor milestones may be normal.

Global retardation = delay in all four areas.

A single impairment, such as severe visual handicap, can affect the acquisition of all other skills. If this is not allowed for the handicap will appear global, even though intelligence, hearing, speech and motor skills may be potentially normal.

Out of synchronization examples indicating a potential problem:

  i Isolated slow speech due to hearing impairment or constitutional developmental delay.

  ii Delayed walking from hypotonia or Duchenne muscular dystrophy.

2 Standing normally follows sitting sequentially and is pathological if an infant unable to sit 'wants' to stand on being pulled to sit. Rigid extension of back and legs is due to a neck extension reflex and a sign of cerebral palsy. Well articulated words but 'nonsense' language, suggest autism.

Variations

1 The range of normal within which a milestone is achieved may be wide, e.g. walking 12–21 months in boys, 10–18 months in girls.

2 Familial variation examples:

  i Bottom shuffling – infant does not crawl and lifts legs to 90° when attempts are made to get him to take weight on his legs, and he then walks late, about 22 months.

  ii Familial slow speech is commoner in boys.

3 Prematures' developmental abilities should be up to corrected age allowing for gestation, and is often nearer actual age.

Table 2 Normal language deviations

	Age (years)
Echolalia and jargoning	less than 2.5
Non-fluency ('clutter', not true stutter)	3 to 3.5
Pitch control (ability to modulate voice)	3
Omission of words ('telegrammatic' speech)	up to 4
Unintelligible due to immature sounds	up to 3.5
Sounds s, th, r are often not articulated even after starting school	

4   Knowledge of normal deviations is an essential part of any developmental assessment, e.g. language development.

Table 3   Developmental abilities and warning signs at ages often used in assessment

6 weeks old

Social	Smiles, coos responsively, elicited, and by history
Hearing and speech	Stills to mother's voice. Startles to sudden noise
Vision	Follows face in 90° arc. Stares intently
Gross motor	Primitive reflexes present. Head in line with trunk when lifted from prone by examiner's hand under the belly. Lifts head for a few seconds when sat up

Warning signs
Failure to elicit any of the above.
Asymmetry/absence of Moro, abnormal primitive reflexes (see cerebral palsy).
Persistent squint at any age.

6–9 months old

Social	6 months: enjoys bath, playing 'boo' (H). Chews on biscuit (H) 9 months: shows objects to mother, pats mirror image
Hearing and speech	Responds to own name. By 6 months 'ma, da' By 9 months double syllable babble 'mama, dada', and understands 'no' (H)
Fine motor and vision	Change in grasp from palmar (6 months) to index approach, pincer grip (9 months). Transfers at 7 months from hand to hand. Mouths objects. Foot regard, no longer looks at hands. Fixes on pellet of paper, follows a fallen object
Gross motor	By 6 months bears some weight on legs when standing, and is rolling over. In prone: head up, weight on hands. Supine: flexes head and trunk as pulled to sitting position. From 7 months sits unsupported. At 9 months: crawls and pulls to stand. Saving reflexes: see below

Warning signs
Absent or slow social responses.
Reduced responses and vocalization, absence of babble.
Any squint. Persistent hand regard after 6 months.
Absence/asymmetry of voluntary hand grasp, saving reflexes; persistent primitive reflexes.

12 months

Social	Comes when called, lets go on request, finds hidden object. Waves bye-bye, gives toys on request. Holds out arm for sleeve
Hearing and speech	Understands some words, uses mamma, dadda with meaning Shakes head for 'no'
Fine motor and vision	Casts (throws) objects, watches them fall Picks up crumbs from carpet (H) Pincer grasp, bangs 2 bricks together
Gross motor	Bottom shuffling common, may walk like a bear. Cruises round holding onto furniture, walks one hand held Pivots when sitting, reaches behind (backward saving reflexes)

Warning signs
No frequent tuneful babble by 10 months.
Holds objects close up to the eyes.
Immature grasp, asymmetry of grasp, and of saving reflexes.
No sitting or weight bearing.

18 months

Social	Cup: lifts, drinks, puts down. Spoon-feeds self (H). Pulls at dirty nappy. Domestic mimicry of dusting, sweeping etc (H)
Hearing and speech	Points to 3 parts of the body on request, obeys single commands. Says 6 words, jargons, echoes speech

| Fine motor and vision | Neat pincer picking up threads, pins. Scribbles using fisted grasp. Turns pages 2 or more at a time. Builds tower of 3–4 × 1" (2.5 cm) cubes |
| Gross motor | Walks well, carries toys, climbs stairs (H), climbs into chair (H) |

Warning signs
Drools, no words. Fails to understand commands.
Absent pincer grasp, persistent casting.
Not walking: consider blood creatinine phosphokinase in boys.

2 to 2 1/2 years

Social	Plays alone, tantrums, demanding. Dry by day. Puts on shoes, socks and pants (H). Turns doorhandles. Uses spoon and fork (H)
Hearing and speech	Phrases of 2–3 words, gives name. 'Naming' games. 50 words+ Has inner language, e.g. demonstrates 'give dolly a drink' on request
Fine motor and vision	Turns one page at a time, imitates a straight line in both vertical and horizontal, and a circle. Unscrews lids. Builds a tower of 6–8 × 1" cubes
Gross motor	Runs, kicks ball, jumps on the spot. Pushes trike with feet (H). Walks downstairs 2 feet per tread

Warning signs
Lack of understanding of speech, no phrases by 30 months.
Unsteady on his feet.

3 to 3 1/2 years

Social	Uses toilet unassisted except wiping bottom (H). Dress and undress with minimum assistance. Knows some nursery rhymes (H). Handles knife and fork (H). Plays with peers
Hearing and speech	Gives full name, sex. Counts to 10 by rote. Uses plurals. Understands prepositions (on, under, behind etc). Asks who? where? (H). 3–5 word sentences (H)
Fine motor	Mature pen grasp, copies + and 0. Correctly matches two or more colours. Threads large beads. Tower of 9 × 1" (2.5 cm) cubes
Gross motor	Stands on one leg for a few seconds. Peddles trike (H). Stairs – adult style of ascent (H). Jumps off bottom step

Warning signs
No phrases.
Persistent daytime wetting/soiling.
Clumsy (motor coordination and/or vision disorder).

4–5 years

Social	Wipes own bottom (H). Eats using a knife and fork (H). Dresses unsupervised except for tie, laces. Imaginative play. Plays in groups, takes turns, shares toys, obeys rules (H)
Hearing and speech	Gives name, address, age. Counts up to 10 by 4 years, 20 by 5 years. Knows three coins. Grammatical speech. Transient 'stammer' from urgency to speak is common. Asks meaning of abstract words
Fine motor and vision	Matches 4 colours, copies cross, square, and, by 5 years, a triangle. Imitates a bridge with 3 bricks, builds 3 steps with 6 cubes at 4 years, 4 steps with 10 cubes at 5 years. Draws a recognizable man
Gross motor	4 years: climbs trees, and ladders, enjoys ball games (H). By 5 years: hops, may skip, jumps off 3 steps. Catches a ball

Warning signs
Socially isolated, bullied.
Unintelligible or ungrammatical speech.
Unable to give name or address (parents may not have told address).

H = by history, otherwise by observation or eliciting the activity.

Further reading

Sheridan M D (1978) *Children's Developmental Progress*. NFER
Lingam S, Harvey D R (1988) *Manual of Child Development*. Edinburgh:Churchill Livingstone

Disorders of development and special needs

Definitions of terms commonly used in developmental assessment

Impairment: An abnormality of body function or structure.
Disability: Reduced ability to perform a task or function.
Handicap: A continuing impairment or disability of body, intellect or personality likely to interfere with normal growth, development, the capacity to learn, and the achievement of normally realistic goals.

Examples of some developmental impairments

1   Permanent and serious: mental handicap, specific speech and language disorders, cerebral palsy, muscular dystrophy, autism.
2   Developmental delay: skills improve with maturation. Examples:

- Mild global backwardness.
- Delayed speech and language.
- Clumsiness.
- Specific learning disabilities, e.g. reading, writing, spelling, (defined as a difficulty not due to poor teaching, dullness, physical or sensory defect).

Incidence of some handicapping conditions

Mental retardation   30/1000.
Severe learning difficulties   4/1000.
Cerebral palsy   2/1000.
Autism   3/10 000.
Severe deafness   2/1000.
Blind/partially sighted   1/1000.

Causes of delayed development

1   Deprivation: determine by history and observation.
2   Idiopathic: constitutional, familial. Affects one field only, e.g. speech, walking, with catch-up later.
3   Mental handicap: many areas, often global delay.
4   Specific abnormality: blind, deaf, cerebral palsy, muscular dystrophy.
    See special needs and mental handicap for assessment and management.

   Always be aware of dangers of arrested/deteriorating development. Common causes include:

1   Abuse/emotional deprivation.
2   Intercurrent acute or chronic illness.

3   Uncontrolled seizures, the effect of drugs in their management.

Unusual causes:

1   Hydrocephalus: structural, post-infective or post-traumatic.
2   Hypothyroidism, lead poisoning.
3   Degenerations affecting the brain.

Causes of speech and language delay

1   Deprivation: determination by social history/observation.
2   Developmental delay often with a family history: frustration often manifested by the child.
3   Deafness: all other functions normal.
4   Global delay signifies mental handicap.
5   Autism: abnormal behaviour and relationships.

Further reading

Hall D M B (1989) Assessment of the Slow Preschool Child. *Archives of Disease in Childhood*, **64**, 295–300

Benefits of early detection

1   Minimize disability, examples: in deafness early introduction of amplification may improve the prognosis for speech; surgical removal of a cataract before 6 months preserves sight.
2   Reduces secondary disabilities, e.g. behaviour disorder secondary to slow speech, by advising the parents on appropriate management, reduces frustration from communication difficulties.
3   Genetic investigation and counselling may prevent the birth of a similarly affected infant.

DEVELOPMENTAL ASSESSMENT

Most serious defects are suspected or detected by parents, nursery staff or teachers.

Taking a history reveals the reason for presentation, whether due to parental concerns (important and should not be dismissed) or professional (parents may deny any problem).

1   Further details of the problem or illness. At what age did the parents become concerned. Is the condition progressive, static or improving? Continuous or intermittent?

2   The pregnancy: bleeding, infections, drugs, and their timing in gestation; toxaemia and the length of gestation, birthweight, difficulties in labour and delivery; was resuscitation required?

3   Concerns in the first weeks often requiring admission to the special care nursery, e.g. hypoglycaemia, jaundice, apnoea, feeding difficulties, needing to be woken for feeds.

4   Previous illness, and the response to it. Medication likely to alter development, concentration; exposure to environmental hazards.

5   Developmental history. Parental recall for past achievements is poor except for smiling, walking, and talking, especially if slow. Enquire what he does *now*. Be precise with the aid of a table of normal milestones.

6   School: days lost through illness or refusal; changes of school. School performance may require discussion with the teacher as well as parents.

7   A family history may reveal abnormal or unusual patterns of development. Neurological and non-neurological conditions in relatives, and consanguinity, to be noted.

8   Social and emotional problems may have great bearing.

Observation in the following order facilitates evaluation

Preschool child

1   Play, spontaneous speech.

2   Posture, walking, fine motor coordination with toys (also tests vision).

3   Performance: offer in turn, showing what the task is, bricks, crayons, colour matching according to the level of ability. Observe understanding, concentration, visual acuity.

4   Comprehension of language; to point to parts of the body, to objects in books on request, to pick up named objects, and carry out commands appropriate to age.

At school age add

Reading, arithmetic functions (+, −, ×, /,) writing name, age, address, short story, or drawing a picture of a favourite activity. These activities also demonstrate his application, concentration, and organizational skills.

Allow for strange environment, immaturity, possible language barrier, and the effects of disability, e.g. deafness.

Sensory testing, neurological and physical examination follow, and, if appropriate, investigation (see mental handicap).

Sensory screening: what to know

Vision

Visual acuity: 1 month = 1/15th adult, 8 months = 1/4 adult (6/24), 3–5 years = adult (6/6).

Incidence of visual problems

Registered blind 1/2500 children. At school entry 6/1000 have a severe defect, and 27/1000 moderate defects (mainly squints).
   Colour blindness: 6% of boys have green defect (deuteranomaly).

At risk

1   Retinopathy of prematurity in the low birthweight <1500 g.
2   Familial squint and myopia, choroidoretinal degenerations, cataracts.
3   Associations, e.g. with mental handicap, cerebral palsy, Down's syndrome, CHARGE association.
4   Metabolic disorders: galactosaemia, Lowe's syndrome.

Delayed visual maturation

Uncommon, sporadic, noted by parents as a failure of visual fixation within the first 4 weeks. May take some months to develop, but normal thereafter. Absence of abnormality on history, examination, or electroretinogram, allows an expectant approach.
   Sensitive periods within which action must be taken for function to be preserved:

1   Visual cortex appreciation: remove cataract by 6 months old.
2   Binocular vision is normally established by 6 months: 'patch' occlusion of a squint or amblyopia up to 5–8 years old helps, though some argue that after 3 years of age it is already too late.

Testing for common defects

Acuity

1   Infants: a newborn should fix on mother's face or a 10 cm red ball at 20–30 cm, and by 10 weeks old follow through a 180° arc. At a year, 1 mm sugar balls (hundreds and thousands) are followed or grasped, but now discredited as an exact test. The objective test is forced choice preferential looking, at variable sized black and white gratings.
2   From 3 years: the Snellen chart is the standard. Test at 6 metres, or 3 metres using a mirror. Single letter card matching tests (5 or 7 letter Stycar) are less accurate.

Abnormal result: 6/12 or worse, or a difference between the eyes of two lines or more.

Registration: Blind = <3/60 in the better eye, partially sighted = 4/60 to 6/24 in the better eye.

Squint

Non-paralytic squints are often inherited, and refractive or astigmatic.
Paralytic: nuclear agenesis, tumour or pressure.

1   Manifest squint: use the corneal reflection test, examine eye movements by moving an interesting small object (not a light) horizontally, obliquely and vertically. A paralytic squint is likely if either eye fails to complete a movement in a particular direction. The corneal reflection remains stable throughout in pseudosquint due to a wide bridge to the nose, or epicanthic folds.

2   Latent squint is detected by the cover-uncover test, occluding each eye in turn. Not an essential test. Hold a small toy at 30 cm from the eyes, then cover one eye with a card or the parent's hand. Repeat at 6 metres with a picture as the visual target. A light is unsuitable as it cannot be focused on.

Manifest squint = a squinting eye that moves to fix on an object when the other is covered.
Alternating = each eye will move in turn when covered.
Latent = the eye squints if covered, and swings back to its original position when uncovered.

A useful test of vision is the response to covering the good eye!

Refractive errors   Myopia can be progressive during childhood, so regular testing is necessary especially in affected families.

Amblyopia   The suppression or failure to develop a clear visual image by the brain due to refractive error, a difference in refraction between the eyes, squint, or cataract. Still rarely identified before 3 years old by which time acuity is usually already permanently diminished.

Management

1   Multiprofessional assessment: cause, severity and remedial action, e.g. glasses, soft contact lenses, surgery.
2   Parents receive counselling, genetic advice.

For the more visually disabled, further management considerations:

1   The severely visually impaired have less opportunity to practise and develop gross motor, fine motor and social skills, and with poor sound localization, show speech delay. To avoid mislabelling, the Reynell Zinkin developmental scales for young visually handicapped children should be used. On average, an otherwise normal but effectively blind child performs at half their chronological age.
2   The parents need to teach their infant the location of parts of their own bodies, and where a sound comes from in space.
3   The child has to be shown how they can explore and manipulate objects

and toys for themselves, instead of having them thrust into their hands, which leads to fear and fisting.

4   Discourage self-stimulating behaviours such as eye poking, rocking.
5   Promote visual attention if noted to fixate on light reflections in a mirror. Use visual lures, e.g. Christmas tree decoration 6 cm shiny ball, pentorch inside a translucent finger puppet.
6   Home visits by the advisor from Royal National Institute for the Blind. A local peripatetic teacher liaises with the schools/special schooling. Sunshine Homes are residential schools which accept blind children, who require Braille, from 3 years old.
7   Learning ability assessment: size of type needed, lighting, low vision aids, need for proximity to blackboard, or use of a whiteboard with black marker pen for enhanced visual contrast.
8   Mobility assessment, and ability safely to cross the road.

Hearing

Normal speech development requires adequate hearing. A loss of more than 30 dB for any length of time in early childhood may delay or prevent this acquisition, depending on severity.

Incidence

1/1000 children are profoundly deaf (usually sensorineural or mixed) requiring special educational provision, 2/1000 are moderately deaf needing hearing aids only.

40/1000 school age children are mildly affected, usually conductive from secretory otitis media, and benefit from being close to the teacher in class.

At risk

1   Parental observations and concerns. Delayed language development. Behavioural and educational difficulties.
2   Family history of deafness (50% of congenital cases are genetic).
3   Child is low birthweight, has cerebral palsy, or a malformation, e.g. cleft palate.
4   History of recurrent otitis, or of meningitis/encephalitis.

Causes of deafness

Middle ear disease (common); exclude wax and foreign body first!

1   Secretory otitis media: post-otitis media, allergy, air pollution.
2   Barotrauma: blow to the ear, pressure changes in aircraft.
3   Facial malformations, e.g. cleft palate, absent/defective ossicular chain, e.g. Treacher-Collins syndrome.
4   Down's syndrome, Turner's syndrome.

Sensorineural deafness (uncommon or rare)

1   Genetic (60%): isolated AR or AD or as part of a syndrome, e.g. Waardenburg.

2   Perinatal difficulties (10%), especially in the low birthweight and premature (asphyxia, hyperbilirubinaemia, congenital infection).
3   Infection:

    i   Congenital (10%), e.g. rubella, cytomegalovirus, toxoplasmosis.
    ii Acquired (10%), e.g. measles, mumps, meningitis, encephalitis.

4   Trauma: injury to the base of the skull.
5   Toxins: ototoxic levels of aminoglycosides.

Behavioural clues: failure to quiet to mother's voice, babble ceases (in some profoundly deaf it may continue for months) or becomes monotonous. Behaviour problems, poor speech development or school progress in the older child.

Hearing tests

1   Infancy to 3 years
For screening purposes the minimum level should be 30–40 dB. A sound level meter, to monitor the voice level, is desirable.

From 6–9 months: the distraction test.
Sounds presented at 45° behind the ear:

High frequency: Manchester rattle, 'ss' sound, cup and spoon around its rim.
Low frequency: 'ooo' or 'hum'.

From 2½ years: auditory discrimination of consonant sounds.

    i   McCormick toy discrimination test, consists not of phonetically balanced sounds but similar sounds: 14 toys in seven pairs, e.g. plane/plate, duck/cup, tree/key, cow/house, fork/horse, spoon/shoe, lamb/man. Each toy is named, the child is then invited to identify by pointing or looking at a named toy while the examiner's mouth is covered to prevent lip reading.
    ii Performance test: Kendal 'go' game at different sound intensities, puts men in boat on command 'go' or 'sss'.

2   From 5 years: pure tone audiometry 'sweep' at 20 dB, at 500 Hz, 1, 2, and 4 kHz.

Grades of hearing loss

Mild 25–35 dB, moderate 40–60 dB, severe >60 dB, profound >90 dB.

Management

1   Assess severity, cause, language development and educational abilities, and any associated behaviour difficulties.
2   In secretory otitis media the use of antibiotics and decongestants are of doubtful value. If loss is persistent consider grommets, +/– adenoidectomy.
3   Counsel parents on behaviour, safety hazards in traffic, genetics.

4 *Even the profoundly deaf have some hearing*, mandating the provision of oral training and hearing aids appropriate to the deficit. Makaton and finger signing are adjuncts, or the main method of communication.

5 Inform the local peripatetic teacher of the deaf, in moderate or severe loss, and the local education authority about schooling needs.

Further reading

Feilder A R (1989) The management of squint. *Archives of Disease in Childhood*, **64**, 413–418

McCormick B (1986) Hearing screening for the very young. *Recent Advances in Paediatrics*. R Meadow (ed) Edinburgh:Churchill Livingstone, pp 185–199

Tweedie J (1987) *Children's Hearing Problems: Their Significance, Detection and Management*. Bristol:Wright

Learning disability (Mental handicap)

Definition

Reduced intellectual function with greater dependence on others for personal and social needs than expected for age.

Incidence

Educationally subnormal, moderate (ESN(M)) = IQ 50–69
= 20/1000 children.
Educationally subnormal, severe (ESN(S)) = IQ <50
= 4/1000 children.

Causes of mental handicap

1 In children found to be ESN(M)

    i Normal variation: at the lower end of the normal bell shaped distribution.

    ii Familial, social and polygenic factors. Children of manual workers ×9 non-manual.

    iii Fragile X in 20% of males.

    iv Trauma, cerebral palsy, meningitis, brain malformation in 5%.
    About 90% have no specific 'pathological' condition.

2 ESN(S): 75% are likely to have a recognizable pathology and 75% are prenatal (i–iii):

    i Down's syndrome 30%, fragile X, other chromosome anomalies 20%.

    ii Genetic: <5%

        a. Individually rare: e.g. inborn errors of metabolism (only 1% of the total).

        b. Syndromes: usually sporadic but occasionally familial, e.g. hydrocephalus, craniostenosis.

        c. Recognizable genetic syndromes: e.g. Noonan's, dystrophia myotonica, tuberous sclerosis.

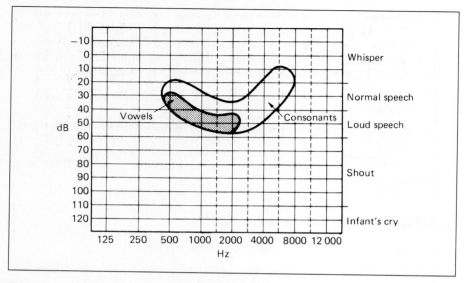

Figure 5 Normal speech sound frequencies, and the pattern of distribution in normal speech (note the banana shape)

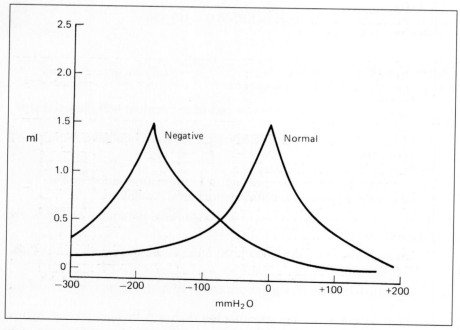

Figure 6 Tympanogram, showing one normal ear and one retracted, mobile ear drum showing negative pressures but no fluid in the ear. Hearing is therefore not significantly affected

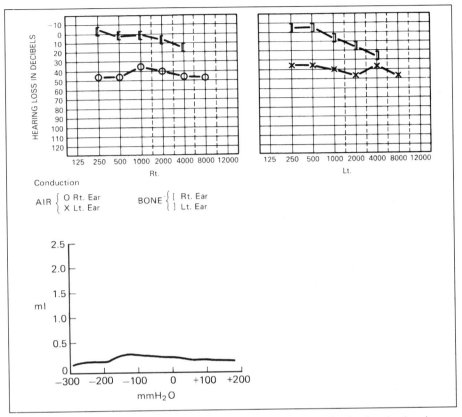

Figure 7 Audiogram. The commonest abnormality, showing a conductive hearing loss in both ears, confirmed by normal bone conduction. The tympanogram has no peak, indicating fluid is present in the middle ear

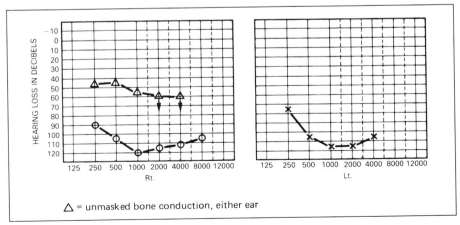

Figure 8 Audiogram. Severe bilateral sensorineural hearing loss. Note that bone conduction thresholds measure down to a maximum of 60 dB. A *false* air–bone gap appears in severe loss

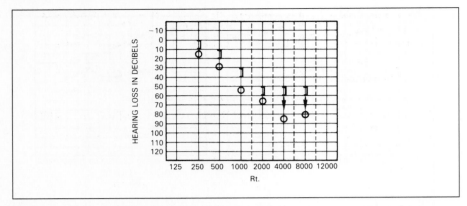

Figure 9 Audiogram. Severe high frequency loss, moderate mid frequency loss 'ski slope' curve of birth asphyxia or hyperbilirubinaemia

   iii Prenatal: 20%, congenital infection, alcohol, drugs, intrauterine growth retardation, structural brain abnormalities, e.g. absent corpus callosum, porencephaly.

   iv Perinatal: 10%, premature delivery, hypoxia, brain damage, intraventricular haemorrhage, hypoglycaemia, jaundice.

   v Postnatal: 10%, CNS infection, trauma including non-accidental injury, status epilepticus, hydrocephalus, craniostenosis, metabolic, e.g. hypernatraemia, hypothyroidism, hypoglycaemia, lead poisoning.

Many ESN(S) children also have epilepsy and/or cerebral palsy, and sensory handicaps.

Aids to diagnosis

Timing of presentation

1   At birth due to antecedent history (ii–iii) or findings (i).
2   Parental suspicions.
3   Detected at follow-up of (iv), (v).

Pointers to mental handicap from the history

1   Abnormal behaviour: excessively 'good', has to be woken for feeds, unresponsive, suspected of deafness.
2   Abnormal motor patterns: floppy/stiff, preservation of primitive reflexes, later hyperactivity and repetitive stereotyped behaviour, e.g. turning on taps, rocking, running in circles.
3   Failure to thrive, feeding difficulties.
4   Delayed milestones of development.

Presence of a good 'handle'

•   Facial, e.g. Down's facies, William's, Prader–Willi, de Lange.

- Limbs, e.g. broad thumbs and toes in Rubinstein–Taybi syndrome.
- Association of abnormalities, e.g. CHARGE.
- Microcephaly and short stature, e.g. Seckel's bird headed dwarf.

Pitfalls (differential diagnosis)

1 Normal variation, familial patterns of development.
2 Lack of stimulation: inexperience, ignorance, deprivation, parental depression, abuse.
3 Sensory disorder: deaf, partially sighted.
4 Medical disease: malabsorption, acute illness.
5 Autism.
6 Degenerative disease, i.e. initially normal development.

Investigation

1 For genetic disease: Wood's light for skin manifestations of tuberous sclerosis (TS), blood for calcium, amino acids, thyroid function, urine for organic acids, mucopolysaccharides if indicated, serology for TORCH, urine for cytomegalovirus.
2 Chromosomes for suggestive stigmata, and fragile X examination in physically normal ESN(M) boys, especially with a family history, or if the mother is intellectually 'slow'.
3 Skull X-ray for calcification due to TS and congenital infection, CT scan for suspected TS or structural abnormality, e.g. with cerebral palsy, seizures.
4 EEG only if seizures are present.

Management

1 Counselling and support of parents and siblings from the District Handicap Team (see Services for the handicapped, p. 24).
Aims are:

- To help come to terms with handicap.
- Enlist active participation in therapy.
- Anticipatory guidance to prevent or minimize difficult behaviour. Identification of a syndrome, e.g. de Lange's, Prader–Willi, Williams' enables more accurate prediction of associated problems, levels of functioning, and prognosis. This 'labelling' may be welcomed by some parents by removing uncertainty.

2 Assessment, needs, therapeutic programmes for stimulation (e.g. Portage scheme), speech, physiotherapy, self-help skills (see CP).
3 Notify Education Authority for instigation of a Statement of Special Needs, seeking parental permission first.
4 Behaviour modification for behaviour difficulties, e.g. head banging, self-mutilation, masturbation in public.
5 Medication: for seizures; in uncontrollable hyperactivity try chlorpromazine, haloperidol (beware of its extrapyramidal side effects requiring an anticholinergic), and the paradoxical action of amphetamines.

Prognosis

1   Life expectancy is reduced for ESN(S), especially in early childhood, due to respiratory infection, seizures, and associated congenital anomalies, e.g. cyanotic congenital heart disease in Down's syndrome.
2   Psychological problems in 50% of ESN(S); 30% of ESN(M) also have behavioural and emotional difficulties.
3   Majority of ESN(M) can be independent, in sheltered workshops, 'niche' employment (gardeners, labourers) in better economic times. Otherwise likely to attend a Local Authority occupation centre, often living in sheltered accommodation. ESN(S) require constant supervision, with the family, or in a residential home or hostel sooner or later.

Prevention

1   Antenatal diagnosis: for mothers >35 years old (Down's), a family history of untreatable, but detectable in utero, inborn error, or heritable brain malformation likely to show on US.
2   Education: dangers of alcohol abuse; avoid delaying child-bearing too long.
3   Effective universal immunization against rubella.

Further reading

Blasco P A (1991) Pitfalls in developmental diagnosis. *Pediatric Clinics of North America*, **38**, 1425–1438
Illingworth R S (1987) Pitfalls in developmental diagnosis. *Archives of Disease in Childhood*, **62**, 860–865

Services for the handicapped child in the UK

These involve health, education, and social services. Coordination is through joint working groups and a statement of each individual's needs.

Health services are coordinated by the NHS District handicap team – a multidisciplinary group of professionals led by the community or hospital based paediatrician, often based at an assessment centre.

The district handicap team's (DHT) role is to investigate and assess children referred with physical and neurological disabilities.

*   The information acquired is pooled at a case discussion.
*   Diagnosis, treatment plan, advice and support for the family are planned and a written record made.
*   The findings and plans are discussed with the parents, and they may be given a written report too.
*   The DHT arranges and coordinates treatment, is a resource centre for information, aids, training, support and advice.

Education

The 1981 Education Act sees any child with a learning disorder as one with greater educational difficulties than the majority of children of their age, or to have a disability which prevents or hinders them from making use of the educational facilities generally provided for children of their age.

Size of the problem

Twenty per cent of school children have a special educational need at some stage in their school careers.

Six per cent of all children under 15 years have a chronic physical disability, and 10–15% have psychological disturbances, affecting school performance.

Learning difficulties increase $\times$ 3 (from 5/1000 at 7 years to 16/1000 by 16 years), and maladjustment $\times$ 8 (from 0.6/1000 to 5/1000 over the same period).

Chronic disability includes asthma, diabetes, bleeding and behaviour disorders, as well as mental handicap, cerebral palsy, spina bifida, and sensory disorders.

Educational need, not category of handicap, determines placement in an ordinary school, a remedial unit in an ordinary school, or special or residential school.

The Warnock report recommended integration into ordinary schools, with special provision, so long as the parents agree and the placement is not detrimental to the other children in the school. The ability to provide from within available resources is the limiting factor, e.g. classroom amplification equipment, remedial help for specific learning difficulties.

A 'Statement of Special Educational Needs' empowers and obliges the local education authority to assess all children notified to them who may have special needs. From the age of 2 years, and younger if the parents request, a multidisciplinary assessment is done. The parents' views must be sought throughout, and a copy of the report given them. If they object to the recommendations they may appeal, ultimately to the Secretary of State for Education. Annual reviews continue to 13 years old when plans must be made for future education or employment.

Social services

Provide: social work support, placement in day care, or residential care; arrange respite care for the family to have time off from caring.

Advise on entitlements for disabled people in UK:

i   Disability living allowance (DLA) from 6 months old, if in need of frequent attention to body functions or continual supervision to avoid danger to themselves or others by day and/or by night.
ii Invalid care allowance for the carer who has to stay at home.
iii Mobility allowance. Aged over 5 years and unable/virtually unable to walk.
iv Severe disablement allowance if >16 years and unable to work.

The Joseph Rowntree Family Fund disburses money for specific items of related need, e.g. washing machine, tumble drier.

Further reading

Blackman J A (ed) (1991) Development and behavior: the very young child. *Pediatric Clinics of North America*, **38**

Chamberlain M A (1987) The physically handicapped school leaver. *Archives of Diseases in Childhood*, **62**, 3–5

Colver A F, Robinson A (1989) Establishing a register for children with special needs. *Archives of Disease in Childhood*, **64**, 1200–1203

NEUROLOGICAL PROBLEMS

Neurological examination

As with developmental assessment, observation of spontaneous activity will demonstrate most aspects of function, and potential disabilities will become evident.

Age, allowing for gestation, determines our expectations of ability to assume body postures, control movements, and perform tasks.

Posture in infants

Observe, place in supine, pull to sit, stand, suspend and then return baby to the couch in prone.

1   Supine: with the head in the midline, look for asymmetry of movement (hemiplegia), difficulty in raising limbs against gravity (floppy). Tendency to stiff extension occurs in dystonia and spasticity, and the child may exhibit spontaneous upgoing toes.
2   Pull to sit: response is graded against that expected for age. Is head lag excessive? and lack of flexion at elbow? (see floppy infants); are saving reflexes and sitting balance present? (see reflexes and Table 4).
3   Stand: ability to take weight is usually present from birth to 3 months, and 'bouncing' on the feet at 4–6 months. Failure to do so suggests developmental motor retardation, hypotonia, hypotonic CP; alternatively, is there rigid extension suggestive of early CP?
4   Horizontal suspension. Normal: arching of back and head above the horizontal from 4 months. If head and limbs hang down, consider hypotonia, or hydrocephalus.
5   Vertical suspension: limbs normally are flexed up to 6 months old. Look for 'scissoring' of the legs in spastic/dystonic CP, or the flexed hips and extended knees of the bottom shuffler.
6   Prone: arched back, extended neck may be excessive in hydrocephalus. Assess ability to take weight on the forearms or hands and the position of the hips, progressing from fully flexed (term infant) to fully extended and rocking on the abdomen by 6–7 months.

Already mobile

1   Crawling: reciprocal pattern, present by 9–12 months? or any asymmetry due to palsy, dislocated hip?
2   Look at, and listen to, the walking pattern (assessment of gait).

   i   Limp: hemiplegia, joint disease, length asymmetry.
   ii   Stumbling, broad based: ataxia, ataxic or dyskinetic cerebral palsy.
   iii   Up on tip-toe: spastic cerebral palsy [CP], contracture of heel cord in muscular dystrophy; talipes; behavioural.
   iv   Waddling or lurching gait: dislocation of hip(s), muscular dystrophy, polymyositis, old polio, peripheral neuropathy.
   v   Steppage gait = foot drop: damage to sciatic nerve, peroneal muscular atrophy, lead, thallium poisoning.

vi Pes cavus: Friedreich's ataxia, spinal cord injury, spina bifida, diastematomyelia, spinal tumours.

Upper limb function

Observation for:

1   Posture: especially asymmetry, e.g. hemiplegic posture, 'waiter's tip' position of Erb's.
2   Accessory movements

   i Chorea is rapid involuntary, non-stereotyped movements of face and extremities, present at rest, worse with stress and effort. Demonstrate 'dinner fork' hands on extending the arms in front, pronation of arms and hands when extended above the head. Causes include anticonvulsants, benign familial chorea, post streptococcal chorea, Wilson's disease, Huntington's chorea.

   ii Tremor at rest: Fine = hyperthyroidism, familial or constitutional.

   iii Action tremor (picking up toys, finger-nose-finger test) in physiological tremor and cerebellar lesions.

   iv Athetoid slow involuntary writhing movements of the proximal limbs in cerebral palsy.

   v Habit tic, e.g. allergic salute of rubbing nose with back of hand.

3   Weakness and floppiness: level may be central, spinal, peripheral nerve, neuromuscular junction or muscular (see floppy infants).
4   Grasp and manipulative skills (Figures 10 and 11). Influenced by maturation, motor strength and coordination, and visual defects. Observe play with a toy, threading beads, pencil grasp and control.

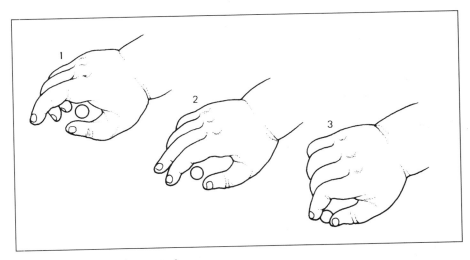

Figure 10 Normal development of grasp
   1. Raking movement at 6 months
   2. Scissor movement between thumb and middle phalanx of index finger
   3. Pincer grasp

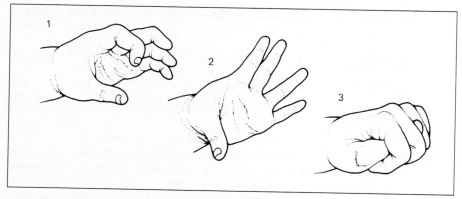

Figure 11 Abnormal hand postures when attempting to grasp
    1. Spastic
    2. Athetoid
    3. Mana obscena, unable to remove thumb from between middle and ring fingers

Cranial nerves examination

I Smell

By history

II

a. Acuity: see Development
b. Visual fields:

> *Distraction*: hold attention to the front with a toy, introducing a second object from the periphery of vision with the other hand, or by an assistant, into each quadrant in turn. Child should turn to fix on it.
> *Confrontation*, in older children, examiner half a metre away, his arms abducted fully. Child instructed to look at examiner's nose and point at the finger wiggled. Repeat, with the contralateral eye of child and examiner covered with their respective hand. The examiner's free hand is used to wiggle a finger, and the child confirms seeing the signal by saying 'yes'. All four quadrants are tested.
>   This method only detects gross defects, e.g. homonomous hemianopia in association with a hemiplegia.

II, IV, VI: Eye movements

> i Observe for ptosis (hydrocephalus, tumour, migraine, myasthenia gravis) and pupil size asymmetry in Horner's syndrome (birth trauma).
> ii Nystagmus:
>   Ocular   = pendular or roving: poor macular vision due to gross visual disturbance, e.g. cataracts, retrolental fibroplasia, albinism, severe astigmatism, optic nerve compression/glioma.

Vestibular = vertical and horizontal varies with head position, e.g. mumps labyrinthitis, otitis media. Worse looking away from lesion.

Cerebellar = increased looking laterally, eyes drift back, e.g. encephalitis, phenytoin, hydrocephalus, tumour.

Brainstem = vertical nystagmus or affecting only one eye or only when head held in a certain position. Tumour, demyelinating disease, or cerebellar malformation likely. Drugs, alcohol and cerebellar abnormality cause nystagmus on looking down ('downbeat').

Congenital = conjugate, purely horizontal, whichever way the child looks. Normal/near normal vision, neurology otherwise normal. Improves with age.

iii Conjugate deviation of the eyes:

downwards: hydrocephalus, kernicterus.
sideways : towards the lesion if acute, e.g. seizure, abscess, bleed.
: away if established, e.g. hemiplegia.

iv Lateral deviation, ptosis, dilated pupil = III cranial nerve lesion.
v Medial deviation = VI cranial nerve.
False localizing sign of raised intracranial pressure.
Involvement also of VII = brainstem lesion/tumour.
vi Head tilt, if corrected may reveal vertical squint.
Head tilt is also a sign of posterior fossa tumour.
vii Corneal reflection.

V

Corneal reflex with a wisp of cotton wool or by gently blowing at the eyes.

VII

Asymmetry on crying, laughing, baring teeth.

i Acquired lower motor lesions: otitis media, mastoiditis, Bell's palsy, trauma, hypertension, tumour.
ii Congenital nuclear agenesis in Moebius' syndrome, includes the VI nerve, bilaterally.
iii Absence of muscle at one corner of the mouth is associated with congenital heart defects.
iv Symmetrical weakness in myopathies is elicited by asking the child to puff out his cheeks, and bury his eyelids.

VIII

See Hearing tests p. 18.

IX, X

Nasal speech, weak 'g', 'k'; testing for the gag reflex is left to last.

XI

Accessory nerve tested by shrugging shoulders against resistance or turning head from side to side against resistance.

XII

Tongue deviates to the affected side.

Bulbar nerves: affected by cerebral palsy; infections, e.g. encephalitis, polio, TB; toxins: tetanus, diphtheria, botulinum; parainfection; Guillain-Barre; phenothiazines; brainstem tumour, myasthenia gravis.

Deep tendon jerks

1   Normally brisker in the neonate. To elicit hyper-reflexia at the knee start tapping the shin from the ankle up. Hyper-reflexia may also show as a crossed adductor response (contralateral hip adducts as a knee jerk is elicited).
2   Increased in decerebration, cerebral palsy, hysteria, degenerations of the CNS, isolated cord segment.
3   Decreased by drugs, in mental retardation, Down's syndrome, cerebellar disorders, lesions from spinal cord to muscle.

Cutaneous reflexes

1   Plantar reflex (S1) is flexor in the first week, becoming extensor until walking at 12–18 months. Stroke the outer border of the foot to avoid eliciting the plantar grasp response.
2   Abdominal (T7–12) and cremasteric reflexes (L1) elicited from 4 months.

Table 4   Time of expected appearance and disappearance of reflexes and their diagnostic implications

Moro	From birth, for 4–5 months. Persists in dystonic phase of cerebral palsy (CP)
Stepping	From birth for 8 weeks. Persists in CP, with 'scissoring' of the lower limbs, as the feet touch the floor when the body is held vertical
Positive support	First 3 months. Excessive and persistent, rising onto the toes, in CP
Asymmetric tonic neck	From week 1 for 6 months. Never obligatory unless CP or raised intracranial pressure
Palmar grasp	From birth for 3 months. Persists in CP/returns in brain injury
Plantar grasp	From birth until ready to walk, about 12–18 months
Saving/parachute responses are necessary for balance*:	
Downward parachute	With examiner's hands under armpits, allowing the body to fall vertically makes the legs extend. Appears from 4–6 months
Forward parachute	Face down, holding the trunk at 45° to the horizontal. Swinging down towards the couch causes the arms to extend. From 4–6 months
Lateral saving	Swing trunk from side to side causes the ipsilateral arm to extend laterally. Elicited from 6 months
Backward saving	Gently allow the infant to fall backwards from the sitting position. The arms extend to the side and back, from 10 months

*Presence of lateral saving but apparent inability to sit is indicative of lack of opportunity or stimulation.

Skin

Look for axillary freckling and café-au-lait patches (>5 × 1 cm diameter) of neurofibromatosis, the ash leaf lesions and shagreen patches of tuberous sclerosis.

Head circumference

See large heads, hydrocephalus and microcephaly.

Retinal fundoscopy

Patience! Best done sitting baby/toddler up or propped looking over mother's shoulder. May require sedation. Dilate if in doubt. Discs are normally pale compared with adults.

Cerebral palsy (CP)

Definition

A non-progressive disorder of the developing brain affecting movement and posture. It is a group of conditions with various causes and neurological dysfunctions.

Aetiology and incidence

1. Antenatal (60%): most CP is due to an early prenatal abnormality. 'Difficult birth is merely a symptom of deeper effects that influenced the development of the fetus' (Freud, 1897).
2. Low birthweight (10%): <1.5 kg at birth have a tenfold risk. Incidence increasing with increased survival of these infants; 70% of diplegia, hemiplegia and quadriplegia related to complications of pregnancy and prematurity.
3. Familial and genetic (10%), e.g. Joubert's syndrome (AR abnormal eye movements, hyperventilation in infancy, mental handicap, ataxic cerebral palsy later. Cerebellar vermis aplasia.)
4. Post-neonatal (10%): infection, trauma, hypoxia often in already vulnerable children.
5. Birth asphyxia. Only 10%. Relatively few asphyxiated newborns develop CP. This accounts for the unchanging incidence of CP of 2/1000 live births.
6. Grading of severity: mild 30%, moderate and severe 70%.

Nomenclature of part affected, and aetiology

Diplegia = legs>arms: periventricular leucomalacia in premature, hypoxic-ischaemic insult (HII) to cortex at the 'watershed zones' between major blood vessels.

Hemiplegia = half the body, arm>leg: congenital, birth injury, HII, brain malformation (e.g. cyst), child abuse, meningitis, prolonged seizure (Figures 12 and 13).

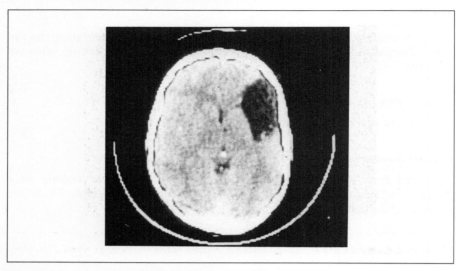

Figure 12   A congenital right hemiplegia with large left frontoparietal porencephalic cyst

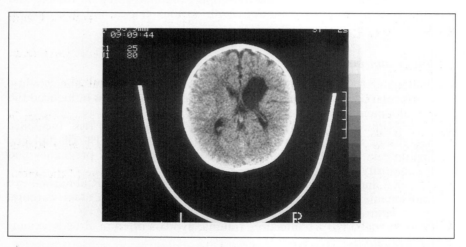

Figure 13   Hemiplegia in a very low birthweight infant with marked periventricular leucomalacia right ventricle frontal horn, bilateral frontal cortical atrophy

Double hemiplegia (quadriplegia) = arms>legs: mainly congenital (Figure 14). Apparent monoplegia (one limb) and paraplegia (lower limbs only) is usually a hemiplegia or diplegia respectively.

Motor pattern, aetiology

Spastic (70% of cases) = increase in tone found in the diplegias and hemiplegias.

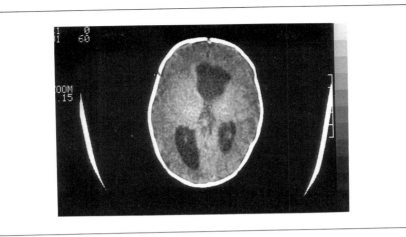

Figure 14 Double hemiplegia with a semilobar holoprosencephaly (a single ventricle in the frontal half of the brain)

Dyskinesia (15% of cases) = constant change in tone: associated with hypoxia, hyperbilirubinaemia.

dystonia = writhing movements resulting in prolonged abnormal body postures.

athetosis = continuous slow writhing movements of the limbs.

chorea = sudden jerky movements of fingers, hands, limbs.

Ataxia (5% of cases) = incoordinate movement, often with hypotonia: in hydrocephalus, congenital malformation of the cerebellum.

Ataxic diplegia (10% of cases) = mixed CP: usually seen with hydrocephalus.

Hypotonia = reduced tone which may persist or precede any of the above motor patterns.

Clinical presentation

1 'Floppy infant' especially in ataxic CP.
2 Delayed motor development.
3 Strong hand preference beginning under a year (hemiplegia).
4 Failure to thrive.
5 Older child presents with prolonged bottom shuffling (diplegia) or gait abnormality, e.g. toe walking (diplegia, hemiplegia), wide based with arms abducted (ataxic CP).
6 Persistent drooling with speech delay.

The motor pattern may initially be hypotonic, and progress through dystonia to a spastic or dyskinetic CP with choreoathetosis.

Preservation of primitive reflexes in spastic and dyskinetic CP – Moro, tonic neck reflex (TNR), palmar grasp, stepping 'scissor' gait.

Reflexes always indicating abnormality: (i) obligatory ATNR (ii) an ATNR more marked on one side (iii) poor arm extension on eliciting the parachute reflex in hemiplegia.

Affected side underdeveloped in hemiplegia: compare nail and foot size on the two sides of the body.

Common associated abnormalities: mental handicap, epilepsy, squint. Hearing deficits are commoner in dyskinetic CP.

Immobility causes windswept posture, kyphoscoliosis, dislocation of hips (especially with tight adductors, e.g. diplegia), and constipation.

Contractures are due to sustained spastic pull, e.g. tight heel cords, and immobility. Lack of physiotherapy contributes.

Investigation and differential diagnosis

Cranial ultrasound for prematures, and neonates with abnormal neurology, has become routine. Echodensities, ventricular dilatation, and periventricular cysts may be predictive of cerebral palsy.

CT may show cysts, or atrophy, often asymmetrical in hemiplegia. Calcification from intrauterine infection and tuberous sclerosis is well seen. Identifies tumour, some degenerative diseases, allows recognition of specific inherited syndromes, e.g. Joubert's syndrome.

Metabolic investigations for degenerations, e.g. Tay–Sach's, metachromatic leukodystrophy and Wilson's, immune function in ataxia telangiectasia, and nerve conduction in Friedreich's ataxia are indicated for progressive disease.

Assessment of disability in activities of daily living, mobility and schooling

1   Self-help skills in dressing, toileting, washing: increase independence or manageability by adaptations to clothes (e.g. using velcro fastenings), and the home, e.g. suction pad under plates, grab handles for toilet, bath aids, lift.
2   Mobility:
    Ability to crawl or walk using rollator, crutches, or plastic splints, or sit in a wheel chair either hand powered or motor driven.
    The DOH can provide special large, stable trikes.
    Assess ability to negotiate streets, board public transport, or drive an adapted vehicle.
3   Educational setting

    i   Pre-school: ordinary or observation nursery.
    ii School: ordinary or special according to child's abilities and local resources. Explore transport needs, access, stairs, adapted furniture, ability to use adapted computer keyboards.

Associated disorders requiring assessment

- 60% are mentally handicapped.
- Squint found in 30%. Visual abnormalities in 20% (refractive errors, amblyopia, optic atrophy, hemianopia).
- Hearing loss 20%. Speech and language are often delayed or abnormal.

- Learning difficulties and behaviour problems are common.
- Regurgitation and reflux with oesophageal ulceration secondary to disordered gut motility in severe CP can be troublesome, and is termed the Sandifer syndrome. Treatment includes H_2-antagonist, cisapride, or surgical fundoplication.

Management

Aim: the maximum independence and self-dignity possible for that disabled person.

1 Therapy
Stimulation of motor, sensory, language, cognitive and social skills equally. Therapists to set realistic goals for speech, self help, mobility, and coordinate to minimize disruption of the family. Global stimulation gives the best results, physiotherapy alone only results in small gains.

Physiotherapy

A therapist's skills are:
 i Advice on handling, bathing, sitting, walking, using transport, and aids to mobility, e.g. rollators, wheelchairs, crutches.
 ii To prevent secondary deformity from contractures, e.g. seating correctly prevents scoliosis and kyphosis; taking weight on the legs using a standing frame helps develop the acetabulae and prevent subluxation/dislocation of the hip and equinus deformity of the foot.
 iii Support and counselling role.
 iv To work with orthopaedic surgeons in planning operations and maximize any benefit from them.

Speech therapy (ST)

 i Help in drooling (behavioural techniques, drugs, eventually may advise surgical relocation of the salivary duct towards the pharynx), feeding difficulties, learning to chew; may use videofluoroscopy for analysing these disorders.
 ii Conventional ST.
 iii Sign language, e.g. Makaton, for the child who understands but has limited expressive speech.
 iv Advice on communication aids (e.g. Bliss symbol board, Cannon communicator, computers) and voice synthesizers.

Occupational therapy

 i Hand skills in dressing, use of toys or tools, writing.
 ii Adaptations to the home, e.g. bath aids, lifts, ramps, extensions.

Portage scheme and workers

Named after the city in Oregon, USA where it was developed. The parents select a desired goal, e.g. to eat using a spoon/dress/build a tower of bricks

during once weekly visits by the lay worker who is supervised by a professional (usually a psychologist). Daily routines for the child and parents are
worked out aimed at achieving these goals by small steps.

2   Medication

   i   For symptomatic epilepsy.

   ii   Drugs to reduce spasticity, e.g. baclofen, diazepam, and in dystonic
     CP some with normal intelligence respond to L-dopa.

3   Counsel, support, genetic advice for the parents. Introduction to the local
   toy library.
4   Schooling: integration into mainstream school for those of normal intelligence. Aids to learning and remedial help, as indicated from the assessment.
5   Orthopaedic assessment of shoes and splints; brace or surgery to correct
   kyphus and scoliosis; surgery to lengthen heel cords, to cut hip adductors in the non-weight bearing child at risk of dislocation from adductor
   spasm.

Prognosis

Initial motor and mental abilities are the most important determinants.
   Diplegias: if still dystonic by 3 years, walking is unlikely.
   Hemiplegias: most walk by 2–3 years unless severely mentally handicapped. Normal intelligence in a third. Seizures are common (50%)
especially in the retarded.
   Double hemiplegias and quadriplegias: often severely mentally handicapped, frequent seizures.
   Dyskinesias walk 2–3 years after learning to sit. Often intellectually more
able than they appear and may be 'locked in', e.g. communication by eye
pointing only. Seizures are uncommon.
   Further education to 19 years for the majority. Employment opportunities
for the handicapped school leaver are limited.

Needs of disabled young adults

Independence through adapted housing, shops and places of entertainment
to cater for wheelchairs. Physically handicapped and able bodied (Phab)
clubs help them meet their peers on equal terms.

Further reading

Scrutton D (1984) Management of the motor disorders of children with cerebral palsy. *Clinics
in Developmental Medicine no 90*. Oxford:Blackwell

Spina bifida

Definition

A failure of closure of the neural tube by 28 days of fetal life.

Anencephaly is the open head end of the neural tube. The infant is still-born or survives a few hours.

Encephalocele is a protrusion of the brain, usually occipital, through a defect in the skull. Hydrocephalus is a frequent association.

Meningocele is a sac from arachnoid and dura elements, contains CSF, but no neural tissue. When arising from the head, hydrocephalus may follow surgical removal of the sac. If it arises from the spine the spinal cord beneath may be dysplastic, with associated minor foot or bladder problems.

Myelomeningocele

Definition

A cystic lesion of the meninges on or in which is the open flattened spinal cord. The commonest form of spina bifida, most are thoracolumbar in the UK.

Incidence

Highest in the Irish and Welsh. In the UK the incidence was 1–2/1000, which fell to 0.6/1000 in the 1980s. This phenomenon is only partly explained by antenatal detection and termination.

Clinical findings below the level of the lesion

1 Motor weakness. Spastic or flaccid or mixed paraplegia.
2 Sensory loss. Anaesthesia and poor circulation result in injury and pressure sores.
3 Sphincter function. Loss of normal bowel and bladder sensation and voluntary control occur if the level is above S2. Urinary incontinence and patulous anus with constipation and soiling are common.

Associated problems in infancy

1 Meningitis. Ventriculitis is usual, with brain damage. Closure of the defect reduces the risk of Gram negative infection, but see shunt infections, below.
2 Hydrocephalus occurs in 80%, from aqueduct of Sylvius abnormalities or the Arnold Chiari malformation which is usually present (cerebellar vermis elongated downwards, displacement of the 4th ventricle and a kinked medulla into the upper cervical canal).
    Ataxic diplegia is the most commonly associated CP, further disabling the child.
    Squint, laryngeal stridor and blindness may occur due to raised intracranial pressure.
3 Urinary tract abnormalities:

    i Neurological.
        a. Absent/reduced function in S2–S4 = weak, flaccid bladder either small, dribbling, or distended with overflow. Some vesico-ureteric reflux but the kidneys are relatively protected.

   b. Spastic isolated cord at S2–S4 = reflex bladder with incomplete
       emptying due to incoordinate detrusor and external sphincter
       activity. High intravesical pressures develop, causing reflux and
       hydronephrosis. Urinary tract infection follows; without interven-
       tion uraemia is common by late childhood.

   ii Structural: horse shoe and duplex kidneys are common.

4   Others: Skeletal: Skull lacunae, extra/bifid ribs. Congenital heart disease.

Management (aims as for CP)

1   Selective skin closure of the defect has come to be considered ethically
    acceptable.
    Criteria for skin closure

   i   Paraplegia below L2.
   ii Hydrocephalus with >2 cm cortex present.
   iii Skin closure possible without extensive flaps.
   iv No kyphoscoliosis.
   v   No other serious congenital malformation.

2   Shunt (ventriculo-peritoneal preferred) for hydrocephalus is usually
    required after closure. Complications include blocked shunt, and infec-
    tion with *Staphylococcus aureus*; if a ventriculo-atrial shunt is inserted,
    shunt nephritis may occur.
3   Urinary tract: monitor function regularly every 1–2 years. Treat sympto-
    matic urinary infection. If persistent, rotate antibiotic prophylaxis to
    reduce the tendency for resistant strains to emerge. If the bladder is diffi-
    cult to empty by manual compression, catheterization is needed to
    preserve renal function.
4   Continence

   i   Intermittent bladder self catheterization from 7 years for those with
       the bladder capacity to remain dry for 2—3 hours. Learnt within 1–2
       days by the child, or parents of a younger child. Soft plastic catheter
       for boys, metal reusable catheter for girls.
   ii Chronic indwelling catheter works well in other cases, provided the
       balloon does not slip out.

    Regular enemas +/– abdominal straining reduce bowel leakage.
5   Orthopaedic supervision of deformities, bracing for walking, selective
    surgery to enable shoes to be worn for walking.
6   Schooling, counselling, education as for CP.

Counselling, prevention and antenatal diagnosis

Recurrence risk of 1 in 20 after one affected child, 1 in 8 after two.
  Folic acid pre- and peri-conceptional supplementation reduces recurrence.
Whole population supplementation to reduce the chance of a first occurrence
has been suggested.
  Antenatal screening for alpha-fetoprotein of maternal blood and selective
amniocentesis have combined with ultrasound examination of the fetus to

reduce the number of liveborn infants to a handful, the result of unbooked pregnancies or parental request.

Prognosis beyond 5 years old

Survival

1 Natural history without surgery = 15%.
2 Non-selective surgery = 50% (i.e. if all children are treated).
3 Selective surgery = 90–100% (about 50% of children are eligible). Criteria for surgery are based on the children found to survive after non-selective surgery.

Degree of handicap

1 Operated on:
   Normal intelligence in 70%. Physical disability is mild to moderate in 20%, severe in 50%; 30% are severely disabled physically and mentally.
2 Non-operated survivors:
   Similar intellectually and in upper limb function to operated cases, provided hydrocephalus is appropriately dealt with, but all are wheelchair bound and doubly incontinent.

Further reading

Brocklehurst G (ed) (1976) *Spina Bifida for the Clinician.* Spastics International Medical Publications, London: Heinemann
Menzies R G, Parkin J M, Hey E N (1985) Prognosis for babies with meningomyelocele and high paraplegia at birth. *Lancet,* ii, 993–995. Comment by an ethical working party follows this article

Spina bifida occulta

Deficient posterior arch L5–S1 is a normal radiological finding up to 10 years old, but an overlying lipoma, tuft of hair, or birth mark anywhere along the spine may be associated with:

1 Sinus or dermoid cyst – may connect between skin and meninges.
2 Diastematomyelia – split cord, with dura or bony spur between the two halves. Traction of the cord on the dura/bone may cause progressive damage as the spinal cord and the vertebrae grow at different rates.

Seizures (see pp. 3–8 for update)

Prevalence: 5–7% of all children have a seizure, but only 5 per 1000 are epileptic (Table 5).

Recurrence risk of epileptic seizure after a first generalized seizure is 50% within a year, and 90% after a second. If focal the risk is higher.

Table 5   Frequency per 1000 and categories of
seizures from the National Child Development Study

Epilepsy	4
Febrile convulsions	23
Seizure with CNS infection	1
Breath-holding, faints, temper tantrums	18
Single afebrile seizure in < 5 years old	21

A close relationship between age, seizure type, prognosis, and sometimes family history, characterize many of the convulsive disorders of childhood.

It is essential to distinguish specific situations, e.g. febrile convulsions or hypoglycaemia, and non-epileptic events, e.g. breath holding, from recurrent, usually unprovoked, seizures consistent with epilepsy.

Febrile convulsions

Definition

A seizure as the temperature is rising from an infection not directly involving the CNS, between the ages of 6 months and 5 years. Duration usually 5 minutes or less, rarely over half an hour and/or multiple.

Management

If no obvious focus, always obtain urine for culture. LP if less than 18 months, unless reviewed regularly by an experienced paediatrician, or if signs of meningism are present.

Prognosis

1   Recurrence of FC is age related: under a year a 50% chance; 90% occur within 2 1/2 years.
2   Risk of developing epilepsy:
    Score 1 for each of the following factors: 0 or 1 = 2–3%, 2 or 3 = 13%

    i   Family history of epilepsy.
    ii Complex FC: >20 minutes, focal, recurrence within 24 h.
    iii Abnormal development or neurology before the FC.

    Of the 0.5% of children who develop epilepsy half never had a recurrence after the first FC.
3   Even after prolonged FC lasting >30 minutes evidence of damage is rarely found at follow-up.

Prevention of recurrence of febrile convulsion

1   Paracetamol regularly as soon as pyrexial. Remove clothing. Tepid sponge is relatively ineffective. Avoiding shivering which worsens the situation.
2   Diazepam rectally once pyrexial, 5 mg under 3 years, 10 mg if older, given by parents, twice daily for a maximum of 48 h.

3   Oral, continuous prophylaxis is only given exceptionally, for regardless of treatment only 4% of the total develop epilepsy.
     Given until 2 years fit free or 6 years old, whichever is the sooner. Phenobarbitone has behaviour and learning side effects, valproate the danger of hepatotoxicity. Drug levels need monitoring. Efficacy poor.

Immunization: simple febrile convulsion is not a contraindication to DTP nor is modification of MMR required, but parents must be warned of the normal response and need for an antipyretic; supply and instruct on the use of rectal diazepam (see p. 4).

A classification of childhood epilepsy

1   Partial = focal onset in a part of one cerebral hemisphere.

   i   Simple: no loss of consciousness.
        Focal motor seizure or focal sensory seizure.
        Benign focal epilepsy of childhood.
   ii Complex: with loss of consciousness, may follow simple onset.
        Psychomotor epilepsy, includes temporal lobe epilepsy.
   iii Secondary generalization: common, start as simple or complex and progress to generalized tonic and/or clonic seizure.

2   Generalized, from the onset. Important to establish it is not a secondary generalization of a complex partial, from the history or by observation.

   i   Absence seizures: petit mal, atypical absence seizures.
   ii Myoclonic seizures: infantile spasms, Lennox–Gastaut syndrome, juvenile myoclonic epilepsy.
   iii Tonic, tonic-clonic seizures: grand mal, reflex epilepsy (photosensitive, sound or touch sensitive).

3   Unclassifiable: neonatal
4   Reactive febrile convulsions, acute metabolic/toxic episode.

Seizures by age (see Figure 15 and Table 6)

Familial factors

Present in idiopathic, petit mal (40%), benign Rolandic epilepsy (40%) and about 30% of temporal lobe epilepsy. Common in febrile convulsions, and when also linked with epilepsy may indicate a poorer prognosis.
     The gene locus has been found for benign familial convulsions on chromosome 20 (AD rare, severe with complete recovery), juvenile myoclonic epilepsy of Janz on chromosome 6 (AD onset in adolescence, myoclonic jerks on waking, other seizures may precede them. Valproate best).

Causes of seizures or coma (aide memoire:A-E-I-O-U, C-'DPT')

A = apoplexy from hypertension, or intracranial bleed.
E = epilepsy.
I = infection:

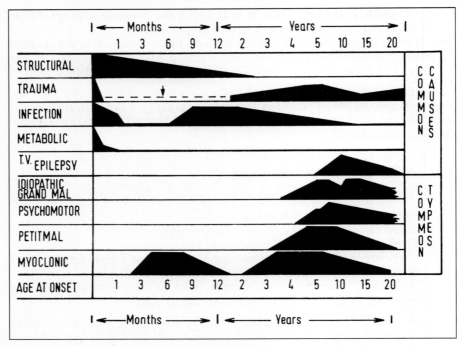

Figure 15   Approximate age of onset, subdivided into provocative causes and types. In trauma, the arrow and dotted line indicate child abuse in infancy

  i acute: febrile convulsion, meningitis, encephalitis
  ii chronic: TORCH, subacute sclerosing panencephalitis

O = oxygen lack (hypoxia) secondary to cardiorespiratory disease.
U = uraemia, and other metabolic disturbances:

  i Transient: hypoglycaemia, hyponatraemia, Reye's syndrome, hyper-natraemia, hypocalcaemia, hypomagnesaemia, pyridoxine deficiency.
  ii Persistent: inborn errors, e.g. PKU, hyperammonaemias.

C = Congenital brain malformation: hydrocephalus, cyst.
D = Drugs, drug withdrawal, brain degenerations.
P = Pseudoseizure: hysterical, Munchausen by proxy.
T = Trauma, accidental/non-accidental;

  i Tumour, other space occupying lesions – clot, abscess.
  ii Toxins: lead poisoning.

Assessment of the child with convulsions

Diagnostic approach

Further differentiation into idiopathic or symptomatic epilepsy follows from history, examination and investigation. Thus, the idiopathic label is a diagnosis of exclusion, and often has a genetic background with a good prognosis for spontaneous remission. Complex partial seizures, on the other hand, are usually symptomatic, with a moderate prognosis and may benefit from surgery.

1   *History*
    i   Eye witness account is essential.
    ii Child's recollection of aura suggests psychomotor epilepsy.
    iii School record: impaired attention +/– performance, in subclinical seizures or petit mal.
    iv Diagnostic pointers to a symptomatic cause:

    a. Prenatal or perinatal abnormality predisposing to damage.
    b. Previous developmental delay or neurological abnormality.
    c. Similarly affected sibling if inborn error/environmental poison, e.g. lead/drugs, or abused.

2   *Clinical*
    i   Nutritional state: failure to thrive in abuse, metabolic or degenerative disease.
    ii Head circumference: reflects brain growth/hydrocephalus.
    iii Skin:

    •   bruising in abuse
    •   ophthalmic division, port wine stain in Sturge–Weber
    •   café au lait patches, axillary freckles in von Recklinghausen
    •   ash leaf depigmented patch, shagreen patches, adenoma sebaceum in tuberous sclerosis
    •   linear streaks in incontinentia pigmentii.

    iv Fundi: papilloedema, pigmentation, e.g. rubella, toxoplasmosis, toxocara; haemorrhages from pressure/trauma.
    v   Blood pressure: raised in cerebral oedema, renal failure, nephritis.
    vi Neurology: assess abilities appropriate to age, note focal signs.

3   *Investigations*
    i   First convulsion: investigate only if <6 months old, or an ill child, or a suspicion of symptomatic epilepsy.
    ii Electroencephalogram (EEG) (Figures 16–22) is diagnostic in petit mal and subacute sclerosing panencephalitis; confirmatory if spike with phase reversal in focal epilepsy, or diffuse spike-wave abnormalities of infantile spasms and grand mal. The mid-temporal spike of Rolandic epilepsy should be distinguished from the anterior temporal spike of temporal lobe epilepsy. If the diagnosis is still in doubt, video + EEG (+/– telemetry) or ambulatory monitoring may record an epileptic event. Note that non-fitting children may have focal spikes or spike-waves.
        EEG is not indicated in uncomplicated febrile convulsions
    iii Lumbar puncture: in an ill child, or after a febrile convulsion with meningism. As the latter sign is not reliably present in meningitis under 18 months, have a low threshold to LP: if irritable, drowsy, high pitched cry, or a rash is present.

Table 6 Seizures by age

Type	Age (Peak)	Frequency (per 1000)	Aetiology	Clinical	EEG	Drug	Prognosis
Neonatal	0–4 weeks	5	Hypoxic-ischaemic, IVH, trauma, metabolic, infection, malformation, drug withdrawal	Tonic, clonic (rare in prem) myoclonic and 'subtle'	Not diagnostic	Various	Variable: see Neonatal problems
Infantile spasms	3–12 months (5)	0.2	1 Cryptogenic (30%) = normal development, examination, and CT 2 Prenatal: tuberous sclerosis, congenital brain malformation, congenital infection 3 Perinatal: hypoxia, birth injury 4 Postnatal: meningitis, encephalitis, trauma, PKU, severe hypoglycaemia	Lightning flexion of trunk, arms extended and abducted or flexed and adducted, often in runs followed by a cry, on waking or going to sleep	Hypsarrhythmic	ACTH, S, Cl	Normal: 30% of the cryptogenic. Mental handicap 80%. Epilepsy 50% Mortality 5–10%. Spasms go in 50% by 5 years, often to be replaced by Lennox-Gastaut syndrome
Lennox-Gastaut	1–8 years (1–4)	0.4	1 Same as infantile spasms 2 Pre-existing severe seizure in 60%	Nocturnal onset. Sequence is stare, jerk, fall; status epilepticus is common. Control difficult	Slow spike-waves at 2–3/s, multifocal abnormalities	V, Cl, S Ketogenic diet	Episodes of minor epileptic status common. IQ and development deteriorate. Mental handicap 80%
Febrile convulsion	6 m–5 years	20–30	Lowered seizure threshold, often familial	As temperature rises, GTCS 1–5 mins Occasionally tonic, focal, rarely akinetic	Normal	D, V, P	Epilepsy 2%
Petit mal	3–16 years (4–8)	1	Genetic, 12% of parents and sibs also affected, and 45% an abnormal EEG	Sudden unconsciousness, no loss of posture. Eyes stare, eyelid flicker, chewing, for 15 s. No postical drowsiness	Diagnostic 3/s spike and wave synchronous in all channels	E, V	Resolves in 90% Grand mal may follow
Benign focal epilepsy	3–13 years (7–10)	2–3	Genetic or idiopathic	Nocturnal onset, half face, arm, may spread to GTCS. Boys>girls	High voltage spike in Rolandic area	C	Spontaneous remission by 16 years

Type	Age		Cause	Clinical	EEG	Drugs	Prognosis
Juvenile myoclonic	10–16 years	1	Genetic, (carried on chromosome 6), and idiopathic cases	Usually soon after waking, initial sudden jerk of limbs and face. Frequently followed by clonic-tonic with brief loss of consciousness. Half have absences like petit mal	Fast 4–6/s multiple spike-wave Photosensitive	V	Spontaneous remission in adolescence
Photosensitive	8–14	0.1–0.5	Genetic, girls>boys May be part of other epilepsies	GTCS due to flashing lights, TV, video games. Usually <5 mins	Photic stimulation gives photoconvulsive response	V	Spontaneous remission in adult life
Grand mal	Any age (6–10)	4–6	Idiopathic, genetic in some. 50% have GTCS as part of other epilepsies	Prodome of pallor, irritability. Forced expiration→cry, GTCS. Variable amount of clonic activity. Cyanosis, salivation, urinates. Lasts 1–15 mins usually. Focal weakness may follow. Post-ictal sleep, headache	Spike-wave or polyspikes. May be normal interictally	C, V, P, PT	Seizure free on medication for 70%. Remission in 75%, after drug withdrawal if fit free on medication for 2 years
Psychomotor	Any age (5–10)	2	1 Scar: mesial temporal sclerosis following prolonged febrile convulsion <4 years old, but see p. 4 2 Injury: trauma, meningitis 3 Malformations: hamartoma/vascular 4 Tumour: 'indolent glioma' 5 Familial 6 Idiopathic	Aura: abnormal/frightening, rising from the abdomen upwards, then quiet, motionless, +/– automatisms, e.g. fumbling, lip smacking, swallowing, looking frightened, laughing, mumbling. Visual, auditory, or olfactory hallucinations. Secondary generalization →GTCS duration 1–15 mins	Focal spike with phase reversal at focus in temporal lobe, or other part of brain, correlating to symptoms. May develop 'mirror focus' on contralateral side	C, PT, V	30% each: 1 Fit free off medication. 2 Some fits but independent 3 Institutionalized care for psychoses, antisocial acts and/or mental handicap. Poor prognosis: Early onset, daily fits, left sided focus, low IQ, hyperkinetic rage. Deaths: up to 10% by 10 years

GTCS = Generalized tonic-clonic seizure, C = carbamazepine, Cl = clonazepam, D = diazepam, P = phenobarbitone, PT = phenytoin, S = steroids, V = valproate

   iv Blood: blood glucose at the time of seizure; serum electrolytes, calcium, urea; microbiological culture, serology, TORCH if signs indicate; for inborn errors, lead level.

   v Urinalysis: blood and protein in renal hypertension.

   vi Radiological investigations

     a. X-ray skull for trauma, calcification, erosion, suture separation etc., abdomen for lead if suspected.

     b. CT: urgent if in coma without adequate cause, or signs of raised intracranial pressure are present. If in doubt, CT before LP. Absence of papilloedema is no guarantee. Structural abnormalities are uncommon if the neurology and EEG are normal.

       A third of CT scans are abnormal in seizures (but only 8% in primary generalized epilepsy) and two thirds if the CNS examination is abnormal.

     c. MRI is especially useful in posterior fossa and spinal lesions.

       Also consider in the 25% with complex partial epilepsy, as 70% of them have structural abnormalities which may be suitable for surgery and possibly missed by CT, e.g. neuronal migration defects, hippocampal sclerosis.

     d. Photon emission tomography (PET) further defines function.

Management of epilepsy

Discussion of relative risks of recurrence and long term prognosis help allay fears. Many parents believe their child is dying during the first observed seizure, and all fear recurrence.

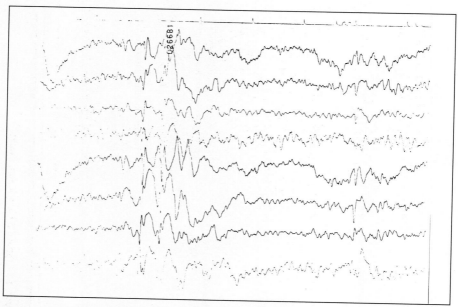

Figure 16   Grand mal

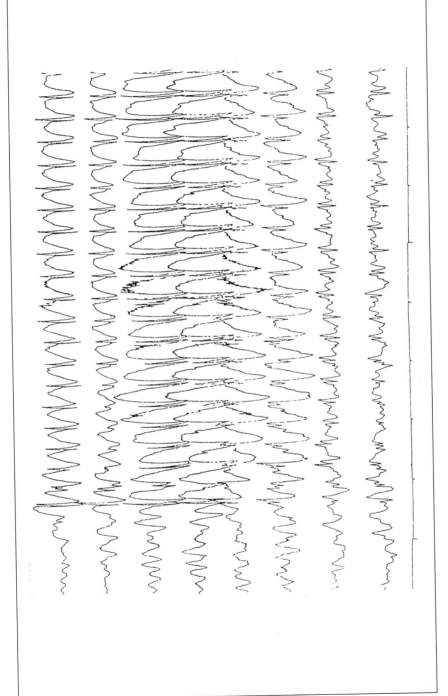

Figure 17 Typical 3 Hz spike and wave

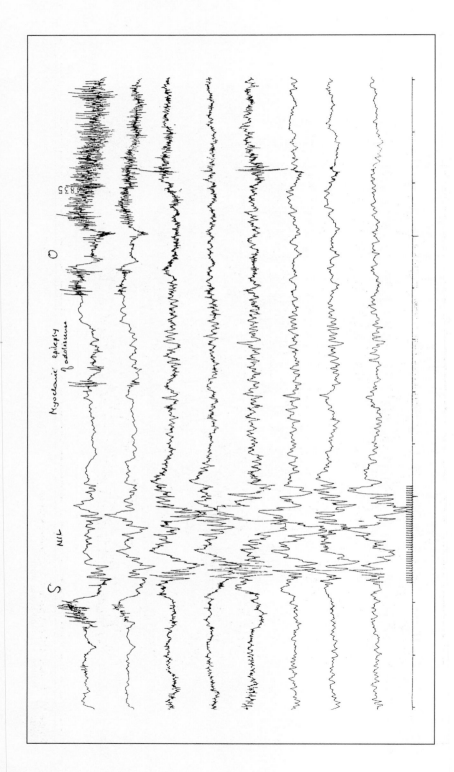

Figure 18 Photosensitive epilepsy.

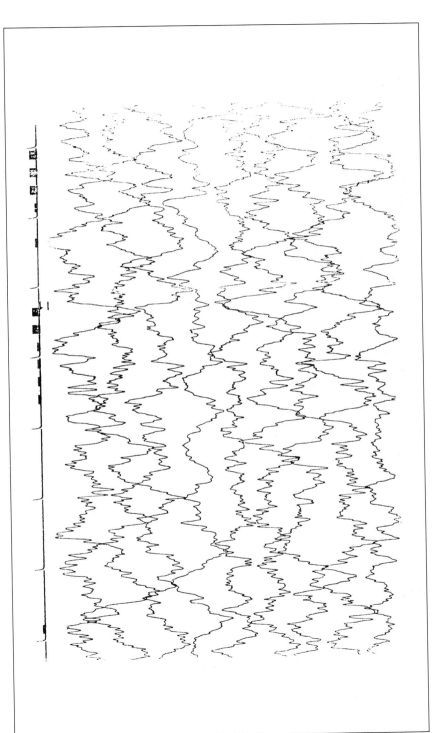

Figure 19 Hypsarrhythmia pattern in infantile spasms

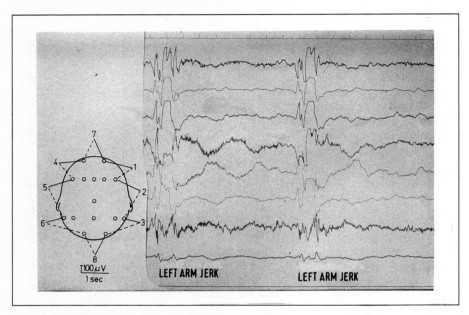

Figure 20   Burst-suppression pattern with myoclonus, in subacute sclerosing panencephalitis

1 Medication

Start after second or third seizure.

Time between seizures <12 months.

Administration once or twice a day is sufficient as half lives are long. Up to 20% suffer side effects.

Number of drugs: monotherapy effective in 80%, 10–15% need two, only 5% require three (or none if no benefit and still fitting).

Progressive regimen if convulsions persist:

a. Introduce first line drug, at smallest dose normally required, up to maximum dose if required.
b. If still convulsing review the diagnosis, add the next best drug, then slowly withdraw the initial drug. Optimize this dose.
c. Next step is to use 2 first line drugs, then a first and second line drug. Once stable consider withdrawal of one of these drugs.
d. Penultimate step is an add-on drug, unless specifically indicated early, e.g. vigabatrin in infantile spasms.
e. Finally surgery.

Special considerations re individual drugs:

a. Valproate often relegated to second line drug under 2 years because of hepatotoxicity (risk 1 in 50 000, check liver function before commencing).
b. Carbemazepine is preferred before phenobarbitone and phenytoin for less impairment of cognitive function and performance.

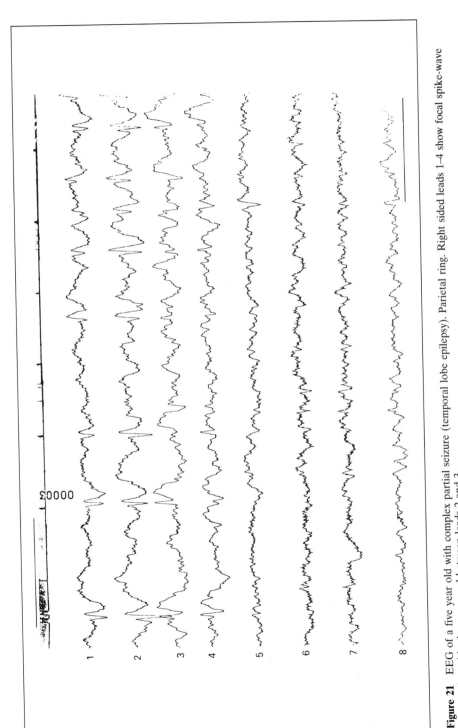

Figure 21 EEG of a five year old with complex partial seizure (temporal lobe epilepsy). Parietal ring. Right sided leads 1–4 show focal spike-wave abnormality, with phase reversal between leads 2 and 3

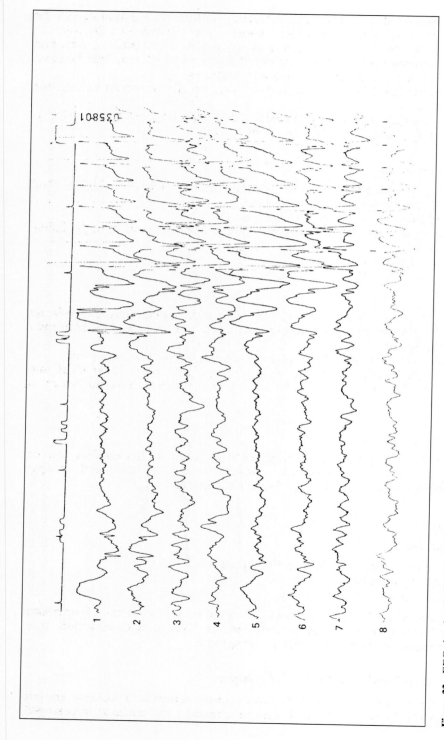

Figure 22 EEG showing focal epilepsy in leads 1 and 2 with secondary generalization

c. Add-on drugs: vigabatrin, a GABA transaminase inhibitor, may be added in poorly controlled children over 3 years old. In complex partial seizures 50% remit, and up to 90% of infantile spasms and tuberous sclerosis. Lamotrigine, a folate antagonist, may help Lennox-Gastaut and other atypical absence attacks.

d. Steroids/ACTH given early may improve the prognosis in infantile spasms.

e. Ketogenic diet, or a hypoallergic diet, may help refractory epilepsy, particularly if associated with migraine.

2 Parental advice

Reassure. Frequently voiced concerns include death during seizure, and cerebral tumour as the cause of seizure.

Avoid fostering an overprotective attitude.

Advise avoiding precipitants, e.g. flashing lights, alcohol, hypoglycaemia, overtiredness.

Give antipyretics for fever.

3 Protection

If fits are frequent enough to warrant medication no bicycling on roads, no rope climbing in gym, and closely supervised swimming and bathing until seizure free for 6 months.

Avoid contact sports. Wear a head protector if prone to heavy falls.

In photosensitive epilepsy, sit at 45° to, and 3 m from TV which should have a back light to reduce contrast. Computer screens have no flicker so are safe.

4 Psychological support

Especially in psychomotor epilepsy where behavioural disorders can be disruptive and attention seeking. Sometimes pseudoseizures and epilepsy coexist, requiring psychiatric guidance on management.

5 Surgery

Indications:

- In partial epilepsy with a defined focus.
- Unresponsive to treatment for >2 years.
- Causing significant handicap.

Best done at adolescence. Removal of mesial temporal sclerosis, hamartoma or 'indolent glioma' of temporal lobe leaves 50–70% of cases seizure free, and most of the remainder with fewer seizures.

Educational and social effects of epilepsy

66% attend normal school. Most have primary generalized epilepsy, and are one standard deviation below the mean in reading and maths at 16 years old.

Cognitive and specific learning difficulties are more common and 34% attend special school mainly for poor educational progress.

Disturbed behaviour, e.g. overactivity, distractability, aggression, impulsiveness, is found in 30–40%, but as it is not specific to epilepsy the concept of an 'epileptic personality' is invalid. Behaviour and psychiatric disorders occur in up to 75% with complex partial seizures. Drug monotherapy may be beneficial.

Poor self-esteem and social isolation are common.

Deterioration over time is linked with continued seizures, and side effects of medication, especially phenobarbitone.

Uncontrolled epilepsy

History of forgetting or repeated dosing is common; obtain blood for drug level (and measles antibody if suspicious of SSPE). If unhelpful, consider CT and degenerative disease enzyme estimations. Exclude Munchausen by proxy!

1　Drug related:

    i　Low serum level. Non-compliance, inadequate medication or reduced drug level due to liver enzyme induction.

    ii　Normal or high serum level. Intoxication from drug excess or idiosyncratic reaction. May be the wrong drug for that type of seizure.

2　Psychological stress.
3　Structural abnormality, e.g. hydrocephalus, glioma.
4　Degenerative diseases: e.g. subacute sclerosing panencephalitis (SSPE), Tay–Sach's disease.

Withdrawal of anticonvulsants

After 2 years of being fit free consider slow withdrawal over 12 months; 60% obtain a permanent remission.

Remission is more likely if neurology and EEG are normal from the outset.

Driving and the adolescent

To apply for, and hold a driving licence, a sufferer must have been seizure free for 1 year.

If adolescent and considering driving, he may prefer to stay on medication. If offering the opportunity of withdrawal, point out that a single seizure counts as a recurrence. Epilepsy after 5 years old bars holding a public service vehicle or heavy goods vehicle licence.

Conditions confused with epilepsy

Generally conditions requiring explanation and reassurance.

1　Early childhood

    i　Breath holding, onset 6 months to 3 years.
    ii　Benign paroxysmal vertigo, onset 1–3 years.
    iii　Night terrors onset 18 months to 4 years.
    iv　Sleep walking 3 years old onwards.

Breath holding is precipitated by a stimulus, e.g. sudden anger/fright/pain followed by a cry, and cyanosis if breath is held in expiration, or pallor if primarily vasovagal with asystole. Limp and unconscious for a few seconds, he then may become stiff with clonic movements, followed by rapid recovery. ECG shows slowing before EEG. Medication is unhelpful. Prognosis excellent. Rarely, Munchausen by proxy instigated by suffocation, e.g. against the breasts, when ECG and EEG slow together.

Benign paroxysmal vertigo is also sudden, pallid, but fully conscious, with vomiting, nystagmus and unsteadiness lasting 5 minutes. Ear infection is a common antecedent. Recurs 1–4 times a month, for up to 4 years.

Night terrors occur in sleep, then waking screaming and failing to recognize parents. Terrified, becoming calm within minutes, followed by natural sleep, with no recollection the following morning. Sleep walk is semipurposeful, and the child usually wakens.

2   Later childhood and adolescence

   i   Hyperventilation.
   ii   Hysterical fits: girls>boys.
   iii   Vasovagal. May be postural or valsava induced, e.g. by vomiting in a migraine attack.
   iv   Narcolepsy: onset 10–20 years old.

Assessment   Self-induced (i) may be a response to anxiety, and not deliberate. Explanation with advice on rebreathing into a paper bag is usually sufficient. On the other hand (ii) is more complex, with apparent loss of consciousness, posturing, +/– jerking, but no incontinence or post ictal

Table 7   Anticonvulsants, dosage, side effects

Drug	Daily dose	No. per day	Weeks for drug to equilibrate	Side effects
Carbemazepine	10–20 mg/kg*	2	1	Drowsiness, dizziness, rashes, GI upset, leucopenia, hyponatraemia
Clonazepam	50–200 μg/kg	1	1–2	Drowsiness, ataxia, salivation
Diazepam	0.1 mg/kg			Respiratory depression with phenobarbitone
Ethosuximide	30–50 mg/kg	1	1–2	GI upset, headache, ataxia
Amotrigine	2.5–15 mg/kg	1–2	4–8	Valproate prolongs half-life; introduce with great care, otherwise rashes are common
Phenobarbitone	3–10 mg/kg	1	2–3	Sedates, hyperactive, poor concentration, rickets
Phenytoin	4–8 mg/kg	2	2	Cerebellar ataxia, gum hypertrophy, hairy, coarse face, rickets
Valproate	20–60 mg/kg	1–3	1/2	GI upset, weight gain; hepatitis in first 1–2 months, especially with polypharmacy in preschool age; pancreatitis; hair loss
Vigabatrin	1–2 g per day	2		Excitation, agitation, psychosis

*Start at 5 mg/kg for 4 days, then 10 mg/kg; avoids oversedation, which can occur even at low dosage in some children.

drowsiness. (iii) Usually occurs on standing still or about to have an injection. Faintness, blurred vision and awareness of falling, prior to loss of consciousness for a few seconds, makes epilepsy unlikely. Elicit an attack using a tilting X-ray table. In (iv) a sudden irresistible sleep urge by day may be accompanied by cataplexy, sleep paralysis or hypnogogic hallucinations. The EEG is diagnostic, with rapid eye movement onset to sleep (the reverse of the usual progression), from which the patient can be roused, unlike epilepsy.

Further reading

Joint Working Group (1991) Guidelines for the management of convulsions with fever. *British Medical Journal*, **303**, 634–636

O'Donohoe N V (1988) *Epilepsies of Childhood* 2nd edn. Postgraduate Paediatrics Series. Woburn:Butterworths

Pellock J M (ed) (1989). Seizure disorders. *Pediatric Clinics of North America*, **36**:2 Philadelphia: W B Saunders

Stephenson J B P (1990) *Fits And Faints*. London:MacKeith Press/Blackwell Scientific

Status epilepticus

A seizure of more than 30 minutes or repeated seizures with failure to regain consciousness between them.

Management of seizures including status epilepticus

1   Stabilize: airway, breathing, check BP. Oxygen by face mask.
2   Establish i.v., take blood for blood count, glucose, anticonvulsant level, glucose, electrolytes, calcium, consider liver function tests, drug screen, blood culture, blood gases.
3   Check blood glucose using stick method. Give glucose 25% i.v. 1 g/kg if <4 mmol/l.
4   Drugs (Table 8)

   i   At time 0–10 mins
       Diazepam i.v./rectal: acts in 1–2 minutes, may repeat after 10 minutes. If fits stop but then recur, repeat and consider infusion of diazepam. Lorazepam is an alternative first drug, and acts for 16 h.

Table 8   Drugs for status epilepticus

Chlormethiazole (Heminevrin) infusion 5 mg/kg/h to max. 20–30 mg/kg/h
Diazepam: i.v. 0.3 mg/kg or rectal 0.5 mg/kg. Infusion: 0.1 mg/kg/h (50 mg in 500 ml dextrose saline)
Lorazepam i.v. up to 0.1 mg/kg, maximum 4 mg
Phenobarbitone: i.v./i.m. 20 mg/kg
Paraldehyde:

   (i)   i.m. 0.1 mg/kg, or 1 ml/year at 1–5 years, 5 ml + 0.5 ml/yr over 5 years
   (ii) rectally at 0.3 ml/kg/dose
   (iii) slow i.v. infusion, 5% solution in normal saline, 0.2 ml/kg/dose

Phenytoin: i.v. 15–18 mg/kg slowly over 20 minutes

Clonic movements persist: paraldehyde i.m. Add phenytoin i.v. to prevent recurrence.

ii At 10–20 minutes

Phenytoin i.v. over 5–10 minutes (with ECG monitoring for ventricular arrhythmias) acts within 15 minutes, or

Phenobarbitone i.v. acts in 15–45 minutes. Watch for respiratory depression, hypotension. Consider intubation.

Paraldehyde i.v. acts rapidly, and is safe if suitably dilute.

iii At about 30 minutes

Chlormethiazole (Heminevrin) infusion for 2 h or more.

iv More than 30 minutes

Thiopentone general anaesthesia for 2 h or more, with EEG monitoring if available.

Prognosis

Most severe in the preschool. Mortality 10%, mental retardation 50%, hemiplegia 20%, subsequent epilepsy common.

COMA

Definition

A state of unrousable unconsciousness.

Causes of coma by frequency

Common

1   Neurological: epilepsy, head injury from accidental trauma or child abuse.
2   Infective: gastroenteritis, septicaemia, meningitis, encephalitis. Parainfection, e.g. exanthema, post-vaccination.
3   'Metabolic': poisoning (alcohol, drugs, medication, glue), hypoglycaemia, diabetic ketoacidosis, acid-base disturbances.

Uncommon

1   Anaphylaxis, stings, bites.
2   Metabolic: electrolyte disturbances, hepatic coma, e.g. Reye's syndrome, renal or adrenal failure, inborn errors (amino acids, organic acids, urea cycle etc).
3   Anoxia and ischaemia including cardiorespiratory arrest, hypotension at operation or postoperatively.

Rare

1   Hypertensive encephalopathy.
2   Hysteria.
3   Neurological: intracranial vascular accidents, tumour, e.g. cerebral leukaemia, degenerations of the nervous system.

Stages of coma

The sequence of progression is reflected in the Lovejoy coma scale used in Reye's syndrome.

1   Lethargy, drowsy. Normal neurology, response to pain and respiratory pattern.
2   Disorientated, delirious. Hyperreflexia, hyperventilation.
3   Obtunded. Bilateral hemisphere dysfunction, e.g. drugs, metabolic, meningitis.
      Posture: decorticate = arms flexed at elbows. Pupils reactive. Hyperventilating.
4   Coma. Midbrain temporal lobe herniation and brainstem compression, e.g. trauma, abscess, clot.
      Posture: decerebrate = extended arms and legs, often asymmetrical. Pupil(s) fixed, dilated (false localizing sign). Hyperventilation or Cheyne–Stokes respiration.

5   Deep coma. Brainstem dysfunction, e.g. drugs, posterior fossa mass, clot.
      Posture: decerebrate progressing to flaccid. Pupils may be reactive if
      due to drugs, otherwise fixed, dilated. Cheyne-Stokes or apnoea.

Assessment

1   History: access to drugs, trauma, infectious contacts. Continue as for
      epilepsy.
2   Posture: see above. Also look for asymmetry of movement, may be
      hemiplegia.
3   Abnormal movements: myoclonic jerks suggest anoxia or metabolic
      cause; multifocal seizures an infective or metabolic encephalopathy.
4   Respiratory pattern.
      Cheyne–Stokes is unusual in children.
      Hyperventilation: blood gases are useful in interpreting the cause.

      i   Central due to brainstem damage.
      ii Metabolic acidosis: diabetes, uraemia, salicylate poisoning.
      iii Respiratory alkalosis: early salicylate poisoning, hepatic failure.
      iv Mixed respiratory alkalosis/metabolic acidosis: Reye's syndrome.

5   Eyes: remember normal fundi do not exclude raised intracranial
      pressure.

      i   Fixed dilated pupils: anoxia, oedema, atropine or glutethimide
          poisoning.
      ii External ophthalmoplegia but reactive pupils: poisoning.
      iii Pinpoint pupils: pontine damage, opiates, pilocarpine.
      iv Unilateral fixed dilated pupil: pressure on third cranial nerve, a false
          localizing sign, from temporal lobe herniation.

6   Motor system

      i   Increased tone, hyperreflexia, upgoing toes in meningitis, raised
          intracranial pressure, hypoglycaemia, Reye's syndrome.
      ii Reduced tone, usually downgoing toes if metabolic or drugs.

Investigations

Blood and urine for toxicology, and as for epilepsy.

Management

1   Establish airway, give oxygen.
2   Reduce intracranial pressure if present clinically (Table 9).
3   Monitor, including the Glasgow or Adelaide Coma Scale (Table 10),
      maintain fluid balance, turn, eye care.

Irreversible coma must be distinguished from metabolic causes, poisoning
and hypothermia.

Table 9   Medical reduction of intracranial pressure

Indication	Treatment
Acute cerebral oedema	1 Mannitol 50%, 0.5 ml/kg in 30 mins. Then 0.25 ml/kg 2–3 hourly or as indicated by intracranial pressure (ICP) monitoring 2 Mechanical hyperventilation reduces cerebral blood flow, maintain $P_a\text{CO}_2$ between 3.3–4.0 kPa 3 Sedation, pain relief, careful nursing to prevent surges in ICP
Tumour, encephalitis	Dexamethasone 2 mg 4-hourly

Table 10   Assessment of conscious level using the Glasgow coma scale

Best motor response		Verbal response*		Eye opening	
Obeys*	5	Orientated	5	Spontaneous	4
Localizes	4	Confused conversation	4	To speech	3
Abnormal flexion	3	Inappropriate words	3	To pain	2
Extensor response	2	Incomprehensible sounds	2	Nil	1
Nil	1	Nil	1		

Score of 3–7 severe head injury, 8–11 moderate head injury.
*Under 5 years old responses are assessed similarly, but in place of obeying commands observe for normal spontaneous movements. Verbal responses are: best response previously known or likely for age scores 5, confused or incomprehensible words, or spontaneous irritable cries if not yet talking score 4, cries to pain score 3, moans to pain score 2.

Head injury

Concussion and vomiting are common. Indications for hospitalization include: focal neurological signs, drowsiness/coma, skull fracture, significant head trauma but CNS appears normal at present.

Beware 'lucid interval', followed by deterioration, in subdural haemorrhage, which commonly occurs in children without a skull fracture.

Management

1   If severe: secure airway, assume neck may be fractured by avoiding head turning. Assess for other injuries. X-rays skull, cervical spine.
2   Assess in all cases:

   i   Consciousness: Glasgow coma scale.
   ii   Scalp wounds, blood/lacerations to tympanic membranes.
   iii   CSF rhinorrhoea, bruising of both eyes or over a mastoid are signs of fracture. Antibiotic cover for CSF rhinorrhoea.
   iv   CNS status: pupils, asymmetry of movement, toe reflexes.
   v   Vital signs: Blood pressure (BP), pulse, respiration. Raised BP + bradycardia = brainstem cone.

3   Post-traumatic epilepsy in 10% of survivors of severe head injury. Onset within one year.

Prognosis

Applying the worst score from the Glasgow coma scale, <3 = 50% die, 4 to 5 show moderate brain damage in 50%, while >5 80–90% have a good recovery, some with minor deficits.

Toxic encephalopathy

Definition

Depressed consciousness, often preceded by fever, associated with seizures, due to non-inflammatory brain swelling.

Pathology

Fatty degeneration of the liver and kidneys is common.

Causes

Most critical are Reye's syndrome and lead encephalopathy. The differential diagnosis is that of coma.

Reye's syndrome

Definition

Characterized by acute liver dysfunction, brain swelling, and hypoglycaemia which may be profound in <2 years old. Associated coagulation disorder is common.

Incidence

30–60 annually in the UK, and declining.

Pathophysiology

Outbreaks associated mainly with influenza B and varicella infection.

Inborn errors of protein and fat metabolism are implicated in sporadic/familial cases.

Some may be due to giving aspirin in the prodrome, and has resulted in a ban on this drug's use under 12 years old.

Clinical

Prodrome of a flu-like illness 7–10 days before, is followed by progressive stages of deterioration:

Stage 1: Vomiting++, lethargy, drowsy, upgoing toes

Stage 2: Disorientated, aggressive, hyperventilation. Enlarging liver, no jaundice

Stage 3: Coma, hyperventilation, decorticate posture (cortex dysfunction)
Stage 4: Coma, decerebrate, III cranial nerve palsy and pupils dilated (midbrain pressure symptoms)
Stage 5: Coma, flaccid, respiratory arrest despite improving liver function (foramen magnum impaction).

Investigations

Elevated blood ammonia and liver enzymes, bilirubin rarely raised, hypoglycaemia common, respiratory alkalosis + metabolic acidosis. EEG changes reflect stages. Electron microscopy. Diagnostic: mitochondrial changes, loss of glycogen. Abnormalities of urinary and blood amino acids and organ acids in Reye-like presentation of inborn errors.

Management

Avoid LP if history and investigations are suggestive. Intracranial pressure monitoring determines the intensity of medical brain decompression and possible need for surgical brain decompression.
Fluid restrict, maintain blood glucose, give platelets and fresh frozen plasma for coagulation defects.

Prognosis

Early recognition (before stage 3) and >2 years old have good prognosis. Mortality 45% overall. Survivors usually recover, some have learning or severe disability.

Lead encephalopathy

Now rare in the UK due to legislation against lead-containing paints. Imported in some Asian cosmetics (surma) and patent medicines. Low level exposure from water drawn through lead pipes, and crops and dust contaminated by petrol exhaust fumes.

Pathophysiology

1 Acute illness: vomiting, ataxia, lethargy, then coma, and seizures, due to free circulating lead affecting the bone marrow, brain, and kidneys.
2 Chronic exposure leads to deposition in bones. Note that abdominal pain, constipation, peripheral neuropathy, and blue lead line on gums are rare compared with adults.

Assessment

Consider any child with

Pica, anaemia, irritability/slowed development – usually precede acute encephalopathy by 4–6 weeks.
Raised intracranial pressure.

Investigations

1 Blood lead level is diagnostic. Urinary coproporphyrins are increased and a useful screening test in an emergency.
2 X-ray of long bones: lead lines at the metaphyses; abdomen: rarely radiopaque flakes in intestines.
3 Haemolytic anaemia and basophilic stippling of red cells.
4 Urine: proteinuria, glycosuria, generalized aminoaciduria occasionally.

Management

Avoid LP. Medical brain decompression is instituted.

Chelate lead with dimercaptosuccinic acid (DMSA), 10–30 mg/kg/day for 5 days, orally (supersedes dimercaprol and calcium EDTA. The latter mobilizes bone lead and may temporarily worsen the condition).

Environmental health officer is involved urgently in identifying the source, and the child is not returned home until it is removed.

Prognosis

Residual learning difficulties, distractability, and mental retardation proportional to severity and duration of exposure.

Further reading

Cole G F (1991) Acute encephalopathy of childhood. In *Paediatric Neurology* (E M Brett ed). Edinburgh: Churchill Livingstone pp 667–699. A useful chapter on mechanisms and management.

FLOPPY INFANTS

Systemic causes must first be excluded as they are the most common.

1 Acutely ill, usually infectious disease.
2 Failure to thrive/maternal deprivation.
3 Malabsorption: coeliac disease, cystic fibrosis.
4 Hypothyroidism.
5 Metabolic: rickets, scurvy, hypercalcaemia, renal tubular acidosis, inborn errors.
6 Congenital lax ligaments: Marfan's, Ehlers–Danlos syndromes.

Next establish the level of the lesion (Table 11).

Assessment of neurological hypotonia in infancy

Antigravity movement is a useful discriminator between central and peripheral causes:

1 Present in non-paralytic causes (cerebral palsy, perinatal encephalopathy and mental retardation).
2 Absent in paralytic causes (anterior horn cell, peripheral nerve, neuromuscular junction and muscle disorders).

Clinical

Lies in 'frog posture' in supine, pull to sit demonstrates gross head lag, in ventral suspension dangles like an inverted U.

Investigation

Dictated by history and clinical findings.

1 Non-paralytic: CT, chromosomes.
2 Paralytic:

  i CSF pleocytosis: polio/coxsackie. Elevated protein alone: Guillain-Barré (GB) or transverse myelitis (TM) or tumour. If in doubt, a myelogram or MRI will detect the latter.
  ii Nerve conduction studies distinguish between GB and TM by slowing in GB. Neostigmine 0.04 mg/kg i.m. restores muscle power in myasthenia.
  iii EMG identifies denervation in Werdnig–Hoffmann and polio, low amplitude in dystrophy, and 'dive-bomber noise' pattern in myotonia.
  iv Muscle biopsy with special stains is diagnostic in dystrophies.

Management

Physiotherapy: to prevent contractures, encourage motor development, general stimulation and for respiratory infections, which may be life threatening.

Table 11 Hypotonia, level of lesion, conditions, and signs associated with them

Level	Conditions	Signs
Central		
1 Cortex	1 Encephalopathy	1 Reflexes exaggerated, upgoing toes; hypotonic cerebral palsy present or may result
	2 Congenital brain malformation	2 Specific features of face, hands, ears etc, enable identification, e.g. malformation syndromes, Down's, Prader-Willi
	3 Non-specific mental retardation	3 Non-specific hypotonia, normal reflexes
	4 Degenerative	4 Initial normal development. Look for, e.g. macular changes (Tay-Sach's), hepatosplenomegaly (mucopolysaccharidoses). Do WBC enzymes, urine metabolic screen
2 Basal ganglia	Dyskinetic cerebral palsy	Dystonia, choreoathetosis, preserved primitive reflexes
3 Cerebellum	Ataxic cerebral palsy	Ataxia, decreased reflexes
Peripheral		
1 Spinal cord	1 Transection or transverse myelopathy	Flaccid paralysis below the lesion, a sensory level present, bladder dilated. Spasticity may develop later
	2 Myelodysplasia	Vertebral anomalies, overlying skin markers, hypotonia, absent reflexes, club feet
2 Anterior horn	Werdnig–Hoffmann (AR)	Fasciculation of the tongue, finger tremor, symmetrical hypotonia, absent reflexes, alert intelligent expression. Prognosis: respiratory death <2 years old
	Polio or Coxsackie	Abrupt onset, usually asymmetrical weakness, flu-like prodrome, CSF lymphocytosis
3 Peripheral nerve	Guillain–Barré polyneuritis	Ascending weakness, absent reflexes. Delayed conduction velocity, CSF protein raised
4 Neuromuscular junction	1 Myasthenia gravis	Transient in infant of myasthenic mother, or persistent. Facial weakness, suck, swallow and cry weak. Neostigmine test
	2 Botulism	Clinically similar, may progress to respiratory failure, even SIDS*. Toxin in food/absorbed from gut clostridia
5 Muscle	1 Congenital myopathy (various types)	Floppy from birth, slowly or non-progressive. Muscle biopsy may differentiate types
	2 Dystrophia myotonica (AD)	Respiratory difficulties may be lethal. Poor suck, ptosis, fish mouth, floppy. Mental handicap. Shake mother's hand – slow release is highly suspicious. EMG ('dive bomber' noise) and muscle biopsy diagnostic
	3 Glycogen storage disease type II (AR)	Progressive, floppy, cardiac failure, macroglossia. Globular heart on X-ray, abnormal ECG. Absent acid maltase in WBCs and liver
	4 Congenital muscular dystrophy	Floppy, progressive weakness. EMG and biopsy, elevated creatine phosphokinase

*SIDS = sudden infant death syndrome

Genetic counselling: for a family history of similarly affected individuals, consanguinity, or after finding an inheritable cause.

Onset of hypotonia with weakness after infancy

Diminished reflexes and hypotonia.

1   Spinal cord

   i   Compression.
   ii Chronic spinal muscular atrophy.

2   Peripheral neuropathy

   i   Guillain–Barré syndrome.
   ii With ataxia: Friedreich's ataxia.
   iii Peroneal muscular atrophy (Charcot-Marie-Tooth).

3   Juvenile myasthenia gravis.
4   Muscles: muscular dystrophies, dermatomyositis.

Clinicopathology

1 Spinal

   i   Cord compression caused by tumours, dermoid cysts, extradural and
intradural abscess, injury, or diastematomyelia.
      Signs: A sensory level +/– hyperaesthesia at the level of the lesion,
localized tenderness over the vertebrae, a paravertebral mass,
cutaneous signs of trauma, spina bifida or neurofibromatosis.
   ii Chronic spinal muscular atrophy.
      Degeneration of anterior horn cells, like Werdnig-Hoffmann.
Usually AR.

2 Peripheral nerve

i Guillain–Barré syndrome

Definition   The commonest peripheral neuropathy.
  A segmental demyelination, onset 2 weeks (1–28 days) after an upper
respiratory/GI illness due to a viral exanthema, glandular fever, or herpes
group infection.

Clinical   Symmetrical ascending paralysis, often acute, also affecting the
arms. Painful parasthesiae may accompany the onset.
  Flaccid paralysis, areflexia, downgoing toes. Muscles painful on palpation.
  Glove and stocking sensory impairment. Bladder may become atonic.
Systemic hypertension can occur due to autonomic involvement.
  Speech, swallowing and respiration may be affected.
  Ptosis, and papilloedema occasionally.
  Often very irritable, and moody for weeks after recovery. Intelligence is
usually unaffected.

Progression   Maximum weakness about 10 days after onset. Recovery
begins 1–2 weeks later, is variable, with relapses and remissions over weeks
to months.

Investigations   CSF protein 0.1–0.3 g/l, no cells. Motor nerve conduction
velocity is initially normal, slowing as the weeks go by. Serology for glandular fever, hepatitis, mycoplasma.

Differential diagnosis Poliomyelitis (CSF lymphocytosis), transverse myelitis (stable motor and sensory level), botulism (toxin antibodies), polymyositis/dermatomyositis (raised CPK), cerebellar tumour (with papill-oedema do CT), spinal mass (local pain, flexed curve to the affected part of the spine due to associated muscle spasm; needs a myelogram). Nitrofurantoin, vincristine, isoniazid, heavy metal poisoning and acute porphyria are even rarer causes.

Management Passive exercises, chest physiotherapy. Monitor respiratory function; if <25% of predicted, cyanosis, disturbed blood gases, consider mechanical ventilation.

Plasma exchange is beneficial in some cases.

Prognosis Full recovery in 80%, not related to severity of attack but to starting recovery within 18 days of onset. Mortality <5%.

ii Friedreich's ataxia

See ataxia (p. 70)

iii Peroneal muscular atrophy (AD)

Definition The commonest inherited neuropathy with onset often <10 years old. Characterized by a high stepping gait, pes cavus, weak dorsiflexion and eversion and absent reflexes at knee and ankle. Wasting of peroneii → inverted champagne bottle appearance. Upper limbs are less involved.

Pathology Peripheral nerves are thickened; demyelination predominates over remyelination, shows as 'onion bulb' on nerve biopsy. Motor nerve conduction velocity is reduced in the common peroneal nerve.

Management Supportive, genetic counselling.

Prognosis Almost normal adult life.

3 Juvenile myasthenia gravis (MG)

Definition

Very rare, autoimmune production of antibodies to the acetylcholine recep-tor at the neuromuscular junction. Neonatal and juvenile MG share the same mechanism.

Clinical

Ptosis, progressive weakness during the day. May be precipitated by infec-tion, or stress. Differential is depression, polyneuritis, and ophthalmoplegic migraine. Neostigmine test is diagnostic. Thymomas, found in adults, are rarely present in childhood.

4 Duchenne muscular dystrophy

Definition

The absence of the muscle protein dystrophin results in a progressive degeneration of striated muscle with fatty infiltration causing hypertrophy. Creatine phosphokinase elevated ×10 normal.

Incidence

1 in 5000 males.

Genetics

Spontaneous new mutation in a third, the majority are inherited as a sex-linked recessive condition. The carrier state and affected individuals can be identified by DNA analysis in informative families, allowing antenatal diagnosis.

Clinical

Late walkers, hypertrophied calves, onset of weakness from 2 years onwards with a slow, awkward gait. Climbing up their own legs = Gower's sign.

Begins to waddle, to become a Trendelenburg dip of the hip, and show excessive lumbar lordosis. Contractures of the heels develop, so he walks on his toes.

Proximal muscle groups affected most, ends up with just diaphragm and fingers in late teens. A third have an IQ <75. ECG is abnormal in the majority.

Management

Mobility must be maintained as long as possible.

1   Lightweight calipers from waist to foot and release of heel contractures with minimal bed rest for any reason can prolong this phase, to about 12 years.
2   A wheelchair from which he can transfer himself to bed and toilet is followed by an electrical wheelchair and total dependence in activities of daily living.
3   Kyphosis and scoliosis are dangers. A spinal brace or spinal surgery preserves the chest shape. Respiratory infections become potentially lethal. Loss of weight heralds the final phase. Death in late teens is usual.
4   Schooling: the level of activity determines when a boy has to transfer to a special school for the physically disabled.
5   Home adaptation: ramps, hoists or adaptation of downstairs rooms into bedroom and bathroom.

Genetic counselling

Of family with taking of blood for DNA studies from the child, female siblings and mother at diagnosis to prevent unwanted sufferers.

Prognosis

Death in late adolescence or early adult life.

Dermatomyositis

Definition

A rare, autoimmune disease with a characteristic butterfly skin rash, violaceous upper eyelids and proximal muscle weakness; oedema may be present. A vasculitis affects the gut.

Clinical

Low grade fever, aches and pains, appear 'malingering'. Dysphagia, abdominal pain, bleeding from upper and lower gastrointestinal tract. Not associated with malignancies.

Diagnosis

ESR usually raised. CPK often elevated, not as high as in Duchenne. Antinuclear factor may be positive. EMG shows mixed myopathic and denervation pattern. Inflammatory cells surround muscle fibres in the biopsy.

Management

Steroids, physiotherapy.

Prognosis

25% mortality without treatment. Now 90% recover, few deaths.

ATAXIA

Definition

A disturbance of coordination and motor rhythm in volitional activities affecting posture, limb movement, eye movements and speech.

Types

- Acute.
- Acute intermittent.
- Progressive.
- Chronic.

Differentiation from other conditions with involuntary movements

1   Acute chorea
Writhing, jerky movements of limbs and face occur spontaneously and interrupt normal volitional movements.

- Interfere with eating, dressing, talking, and writing and cause clumsiness, with consequent 'getting into trouble' at home and at school.
- Increased by emotion, disappear in sleep.
- Weakness. Marked hypotonia with characteristic 'dinner forking'.
- Normal tendon reflexes.
- Mood very labile.
- Duration 2–3 months, may recur.

2   Others: chorea is not usually difficult to distinguish from tics (which can be demonstrated at will), the obscenities uttered in Gilles de la Tourette syndrome, and progressive conditions like Wilson's disease, or Huntingdon's chorea (family history).
3   Drug induced extrapyramidal reactions may confuse unless a history of ingestion is obtained (e.g. metaclopramide, haloperidol, chlorpromazine). Diphenhydramine reverses these effects.

Acute ataxia

1   Intoxication: phenytoin, piperazine ('worm wobble'), alcohol, DDT, lead.
2   Acute cerebellar ataxia: 1–5 years old, post chickenpox, during Coxsackie, Echo, polio, infectious mononucleosis, mycoplasma. Sudden onset, ataxia + hypotonia, lasts 1–8 weeks, recovery is complete. CSF may show up to 100 lymphocytes.
3   Myoclonic encephalopathy: dancing eyes, myoclonic jerking of face, limbs. Present at rest, thus differs from cerebellar ataxia. Most cases are idiopathic, or post coryzal, and rarely an occult neuroblastoma. Response to ACTH may be dramatic. Mild mental retardation ensues in 50%.

    Investigation: requires urinary homovanillic acid and vanillyl mandelic acid estimation, US or body CT looking for suprarenal calcification, skeletal survey, chest X-ray, bone marrow.

Acute intermittent ataxia

Causes

1 Seizure: minor epileptic status, and post ictally.
2 Benign paroxysmal vertigo: see conditions confused with epilepsy.
3 Migraine: basilar type with loss of vision or flashing lights, tinnitus, slurred speech.
4 Metabolic, all very rare AR conditions:

- Arginosuccinic acidura: urea cycle defect → ataxia, mental retardation, fragile hair.
- Hartnup's disease: tryptophan transport defect → mental disturbance and retardation, double vision, pellagra-like rash. Give nicotinamide.
- Maple syrup urine disease.

Progressive ataxia

1 Posterior fossa tumours

Headache, vomiting, head tilt, neck stiffness, papilloedema common.
Fits are *rare*; 55% of all childhood tumours are infratentorial. Exclude Chiari malformation, or a cyst by CT. No LP!

Clinical signs relating to tumour sites

i Cerebellar astrocytoma gives unilateral ataxic signs, with falling to or veering to the affected side.
ii Medulloblastoma is midline in the roof of the 4th ventricle → early obstructive hydrocephalus, trunk and limb ataxia, with a tendency to fall forward or back.
iii Ependymoma arises from the floor of the 4th ventricle. Early hydrocephalus. Infiltrative, with cranial nerve palsies and stiff neck.

Management

Surgery may cure a cerebellar astrocytoma, but medulloblastoma cannot be completely removed and needs irradiation; 5 year survival 40%. Ependymoma less malignant than medulloblastoma.

2 Posterior fossa subdural or epidural collection, cerebellar abscess

Urgent recognition alters prognosis. Occurs after trauma or failure to respond to antibiotics, and a CT is needed.

3 Friedreich's ataxia (AR)

Definition

A degeneration of the spinal cord dorsal columns and cerebellum. Ataxia, loss of position and vibration sense, areflexia, and scoliosis result. Sensory nerve conduction velocity is reduced, whereas motor nerve conduction velocity is usually normal.

Progression

Onset usually in late childhood, with loss of ability to walk from adolescence onwards. Diabetes mellitus and cardiomyopathy appear in adult life, the latter causing early death.

4   *Metabolic (all rare)*

Abetalipoproteinaemia, ataxia-telangiectasia, Refsum's syndrome: AR, phytanic acid oxidase deficiency → onset 4–7 years old, loss of appetite, ataxia, dry scaly skin, progressive deafness, retinitis, peripheral neuropathy. Diet low in phytates is beneficial.

Chronic ataxia

1   *Ataxic cerebral palsy*

See cerebral palsy

2   *Hydrocephalus*

Pathophysiology

Obstruction, overproduction, or failure of absorption of CSF.

  i Obstruction to CSF pathways at foramen of Munro, 3rd ventricle, aqueduct of Sylvius, or foramina of the 4th ventricle, caused by:

    a. Congenital malformations
Aqueduct stenosis: sporadic, or rarely X-linked.
Arnold–Chiari malformation of downward elongation of cerebellar tonsils through the foramen magnum, and frequently associated with spina-bifida.
Dandy–Walker syndrome: 4th ventricle outlets absent → massive ballooning, with a large posterior fossa, evident clinically or on skull X-ray.

    b. Inflammatory disease: congenital cytomegalovirus or toxoplasmosis infection, meningitis, intraventricular/intracranial bleeds, TB.

    c. Tumours: see Progressive ataxias.

  ii Overproduction of CSF: very rare, due to choroid papilloma.
  iii Failure of CSF absorption by the arachnoid granulations: 'gumming up' after bleeds or infection also occurs, but the main mechanism is obstruction.

Symptoms

Vomiting, headache (see below), failure to thrive, drowsiness, shrill cry, developmental delay (especially motor), or mental regression which can be severe.

'Cocktail party' personality = facile social manner and an acquired stock of phrases, appearing more intelligent than is the case. May be found in the spina-bifida with a shunt.

Clinical

- Large head, failure of anterior fontanelle to close and wide sutures (or sprung if acquired after infancy). Percuss lightly holding the child's head with the other hand immediate opposite to feel a vibration or fluid thrill.
- Distended scalp veins.
- Bulging fontanelle – its absence is not a reliable sign.
- Sunsetting sign, lid retraction.
- Eyes: papilloedema is unusual in infants; retinal haemorrhages appear if acute, and optic atrophy if long standing; presence of choroidoretinitis in congenital infection.
- Ataxia: titubation of head, unsteady trunk, intention tremor, staggering gait, hypotonia and hyporeflexia.
- Ataxic cerebral palsy in some cases: hypotonia with increased reflexes upgoing toes.
- Acute signs: slow pulse rate, elevated BP, slow irregular respirations.

Differential diagnosis of a large head

1   Is the CNS normal? If so, is it

   i   Normal variation.
   ii Familial (measure parents' and siblings' heads).
   iii Disproportionate growth in a premature, failure to thrive, rickets, achondroplasia, or haematological disease, e.g. sickle cell or thalassaemia.

2   Abnormal CNS present.

   i   Hydrocephalus, subdural haemorrhage or effusion must be differentiated, by US if the fontanelle is still open, or by CT.
   ii Abnormal boat-shape in craniostenosis of the sagittal suture (seen on X-ray) with minimal CNS signs.
   iii Cerebral glioma is likely to have localizing signs (see below), identified by CT.
   iv Megaencephaly may be idiopathic or due to neurofibromatosis, inborn errors such as mucopolysaccharidoses or Tay–Sach's disease.
   v   Sotos syndrome presents as developmental slowness, high forehead, large hands and feet, initially tall for age +/– precocious puberty.

Management

- Conservative treatment with observation or isosorbide as long as no significant mental deterioration, onset of stridor, or visual impairment, occurs. Intracranial pressure monitoring is rarely needed to clarify.

- Surgery is dependent on the rate of increase, and underlying cause, e.g. a high CSF protein (>1 g/l) will cause a shunt to block. In tumours consider removal, or palliation with a shunt alone.
- Commonest shunt used now is ventriculoperitoneal. Major danger is infection (*Staph. aureus*), usually acquired at the time of insertion.

MICROCEPHALY

Prenatal onset: small head at birth – congenital infection, alcohol, syndromes.
  Progressive failure to grow: postnatal, e.g. cerebral hypoxia/injury, post-meningitis, craniostenosis.

DEGENERATIONS OF THE CNS

Most die in childhood.
  Rare except for HIV.
  Presentations variable, may include all or some of the following:

  Poliodystrophy: Grey matter involvement = personality changes, seizures and early onset of dementia (e.g. Tay-Sachs, Neimann-Pick, Gaucher's disease).
  Leucodystrophy: White matter involvement = cortical blindness, deafness, motor skills impaired through weakness or spasticity, ataxia, peripheral neuropathy (e.g. metachromatic leucodystrophy, Schilder's disease):

1   Eye signs: cloudy corneas in mucopolysaccharidoses; cherry red spot in Tay–Sachs and Neimann–Pick disease; optic atrophy in leucodystrophies.
2   Organomegaly, e.g. large liver and tongue in some glycogenoses; liver, spleen and bones in mucopolysaccharidoses (MPS); liver and spleen in Gaucher's disease.

Causes of CNS degeneration

1   *Metabolic*: a variety of storage disorders due to:
    i   Absence of lysosomal enzymes, e.g.

        a. Leucodystrophies: aryl sulphatase = metachromatic leucodystrophy.
        b. Poliodystrophy: hexosaminidase A = Tay–Sachs disease, sphingomyelinase = Neimann–Pick.

    ii Abnormal copper metabolism, e.g. Wilson's disease AR, Menkes syndrome XL: kinky sparse hair, fits, low serum copper and caeruloplasmin.
    iii Presently unknown, e.g. Huntingdon's chorea.

2   *Infection*: HIV, subacute sclerosing panencephalitis (SSPE) post measles.
3   *Immune disorder*: ataxia-telangiectasia AR.
4   Sex associated.

    i   Sporadic: Rett's syndrome = girls only, regression at 1 year old, hyperventilation episodes, hand wringing, jerks, seizures, spastic CP by 4 years.
    ii XL: Lesch–Nyhan syndrome.

Investigations

1   Urinary amino acids, dermatan and heparan sulphate (MNPS).
2   Blood for white cell enzyme studies (e.g. Neimann–Pick), hexosaminidases (e.g. Tay–Sachs), uric acid (e.g. Lesch–Nyhan syndrome), caeruloplasmin (e.g. Wilson's), HIV antibody.
3   CSF: measles antibodies for SSPE.
4   Bone marrow aspirate: abnormal cells of Gaucher's, Neimann–Pick.

5 Liver biopsy, muscle biopsy: glycogen storage disorder.
6 Skin fibroblast culture: various inborn errors of metabolism detected.
7 Electrical tests: EEG burst-suppression pattern is characteristic in SSPE. Motor nerve conduction velocity and visual evoked responses reduced in some leucodystrophies. Electroretinogram responses reduced in poliodystrophies.
8 MRI: demyelination in leucodystrophies well shown.

Genetic counselling

Most conditions are AR, some AD (e.g. Huntingdon's), rarely X-linked (e.g. Lesch–Nyhan). Accurate diagnosis is therefore essential.

Fetal studies: chorionic villus biopsy for DNA studies (e.g. Huntingdon's), for enzyme testing and fetal sexing.

Blood testing for carrier state, e.g. Tay–Sachs, allows siblings to be counselled.

Management

1 Bone marrow in MPS, zidovudine in AIDS. Gene therapy may be possible for other degenerations in the future, but at present none is available.
2 Counselling family. Parent support groups/societies.
3 Activities and goals depend on the age of onset and rate of deterioration.
4 Respite/hospice care.

Prevention

1 Safer sex.
2 Immunization: SSPE is rare after measles vaccination.
3 Premarital counselling in at risk groups, e.g. Ashkenazi Jews and Tay–Sachs.
4 Antenatal diagnosis.

HEADACHE

Major causes

1   Acute: infection, hypertension.
2   Neurological: migraine, raised intracranial pressure, post-traumatic, intracranial bleed.
3   Tension.
4   Local: sinusitis, dental caries.

Migraine and tension headaches

Recurrent headaches affect 15–20% of children, peak incidence 12 years.

Migraine

Definition

Headache with two of the following: unilateral headache, visual aura, nausea or vomiting, family history.

Prevalence

3% of children, 10% of adolescents.

Pathophysiology

Hypotheses:

    i Vascular vasoconstriction (aura) followed by vasodilatation (headache).
    ii Primary neurogenic (spreading depression of Leao).

Neither is confirmed as the primary mechanism.

Clinical

Onset from 2 years old, may appear as pallor and vomiting alone, and only later is headache verbalized by the child. Other manifestations include recurrent abdominal pain, and slurred speech and ataxia in basilar artery migraine.

Examination

Café-au-lait patches for neurofibromatosis, press over sinuses to elicit tenderness of sinusitis. Teeth for caries.

Cranial nerves, especially visual fields; fundoscopy; auscultation over skull and eyes for bruit from arterio-venous malformation/aneurysm.

General examination must include blood pressure, and if abuse is suspected, the genitals.

Table 12 Migraine and tension headache differences

	Migraine	*Tension*
Character	Throbbing	Sharp, or dull ache
Site	Hemicranial, bifrontal	Often generalized, vertex, or unclear
Frequency	Paroxysmal or isolated attacks at intervals	Continuous or many hours every day for days/weeks/months at a time
Aura	Eyes – spots, scotoma, bright light. Ears – tinnitus	None
Associations	Nausea, vomiting, photophobia	Dizziness, depression, light headed
Neurological symptoms and signs	Transient ataxia, 'pins and needles' hemiplegias, aphasia, dysarthria, ophthalmoplegia	Normal
Preference	Lie down in a dark quiet room	Continue normal activities
Family history	Migraine, car sickness	Not usual
Precipitants	Frequent: hunger, exercise, foods*, acute stress, sunlight, perfumes	Frequently denied, schooling/family problems
Sleep	May wake child from sleep	Prevents sleep occasionally
Medication	Paracetamol; if nausea and vomiting add metoclopramide. If very severe: sumatriptan	Ineffective

*Foods include: oranges, chocolate, cheese, yoghurt, colourings, preservatives.

Differential diagnostic points

1 Migraine from tension (see Table 12).
2 Sinusitis always has rhinorrhoea.
3 Raised intracranial pressure headache is worse lying down, coughing or straining, and associated with early morning waking.
4 Facial muscles tensed due to refractory error (eye testing has usually already been done!) and dental malocclusion with pain at meal times.

Investigation

Not warranted if normal examination and diagnosis is clear-cut. Indications for further investigations (after Hockaday J M (1990). Management of Migraine. *Archives of Disease in Childhood*, **65**, 1174–1176):

1 Inappropriately large head in a preschool child.
2 New neurological symptoms or physical signs. Increase in frequency and severity of headaches.
3 Failure

   i to return to full normal health between attacks
   ii of simple analgesia to relieve headache.

4 Deterioration: in developmental progress or growth velocity; personality or behavioural changes.

Management

1   Reassure. If tension headache, gently probe for causation. If incapacitating or associated with school refusal, child psychiatric involvement is helpful.
2   Medication: paracetamol is safe, and ergotamine may be used over 12 years of age, but is replaced by sumatriptan, a highly selective 5HT agonist. Vomiting can be troublesome if persistent so try prochlorperazine 250 µg/kg 2 or 3 times daily. Although useful metoclopramide in the preschool child can cause severe extrapyramidal reactions.

Prophylaxis in migraine

1   Avoid stressful situations.
2   Avoid precipitants. Dietary manipulation; trial of the hypoallergic diet if severe/hemiplegic migraine.
3   Medication if >2 attacks per month: flunarazine (a class 4 calcium channel blocker) is promising (not available in UK at present). Little better than placebo are pizotifen (0.5–1.5 mg daily) or propranolol (1–2 mg/kg/day), but worth a trial for 2–3 months, by which time the headaches may have remitted.

Prognosis

Tendency to recur for 2–4 years, then remit up to adult life.

Further reading

Barlow C F (1984) *Headaches and Migraines in Children*. Spastics International Medical Publications. Oxford: Blackwell
Hockaday J M (ed) (1988) *Migraine in Children*. London: Butterworth

RAISED INTRACRANIAL PRESSURE

Causes

Within the confines of the skull, too much blood, tissue (tumour, abscess) or CSF. In the relatively pliable child's skull the sutures widen or are 'sprung', thus signs appear relatively later than in the adult.

Rapid rise as with bleed/trauma/malignant tumour or abscess leads to more severe manifestations.

Clinical

1 Headache

Vertex or frontal, worse on lying down, relieved by vomiting. Present at night, on waking, ease up after breakfast; mild and sporadic to begin with. Crying and coughing raise pressure, so both are avoided.

2 Other symptoms

Vomiting may be projectile, and without headache is unlikely to be due to raised pressure.

Drowsiness is a feature of rapidly rising pressure.

Convulsions are unusual at presentation, unlike adult.

3 Signs

Absence of papilloedema is no guarantee.
  i False localizing signs:
      a. Third nerve palsy (dilating pupil, followed by ptosis, divergent squint) with contralateral hemiplegia in uncal herniation syndrome due to temporal lobe swelling.
      b. Sixth nerve palsy due to its long intracranial course, and, rarely the seventh cranial nerve.

  ii Bradycardia, hypertension, stridor/Cheyne–Stokes respiration.
  iii Neurological patterns: see Coma and Reye's syndrome.

INTRACRANIAL TUMOURS

Second commonest malignancy of childhood.

Peak age 5–9 years, mainly infratentorial; rare under 1 year when half are supratentorial. Brain secondaries from other sites are rare.

Sites: 45% cerebellar, 25% cerebrum, 10% ependymomas, 10% brainstem, 10% midline, e.g. craniopharyngioma, pituitary, optic nerve.

Pathology

Gliomas (75%)

Tumours of glial (supportive) cells. Medulloblastoma (see ataxia) is rapidly growing, made up of small round cells. Gliomas of brainstem and pons are also rapidly growing, whereas those of the optic pathways are usually associated with von Recklinghausen's disease and are slow growing with a good prognosis.

Astrocytomas (20%)

Astrocytes are usually benign and slow growing, infiltrative, with a tendency to become cystic.

Craniopharyngioma (rare)

Derived from squamous cells of Rathke's pouch, i.e. a developmental, slow-growing benign tumour producing its effects by compression.

Clinical

Principal symptoms and signs are the result of three mechanisms:

1   Raised intracranial pressure.
2   Brain shifts.
3   Local infiltration.

Signs

- Hydrocephalus: bulging fontanelle, or if sutures are already fused, a 'cracked pot' note on skull percussion.
- Cerebellar involvement:

  Unilateral – incoordination on the same side.
  Midline   – incoordination both sides. Signs are intention or action tremor, dysdiadokokinesis, unsteady gait, hypotonia, hyporeflexia, nystagmus, slow dysrhythmic speech.

- Occiput tilted to the side of the tumour due to nerve traction or to correct a strabismus from a sixth nerve palsy.
- Stiffness and neck pain.

- Cranial nerve palsies: infiltration (brainstem gliomas) pressure effects producing false localizing signs (cerebellar astrocytomas).
- Pituitary abnormalities, visual field defects, optic atrophy in craniopharyngioma, optic nerve gliomas. The latter also presents with unilateral or asymmetrical nystagmus.
- Focal seizures in supratentorial gliomas: a rare cause of local seizures in childhood, but must be considered if they are intractable or hemiplegia develops.
- Seeding in medulloblastoma and brainstem glioma → cord compression with paraplegia/spinal nerve root infiltration with root pains, areflexia, spinal tenderness.

Investigation

Skull X-ray may show pressure effects: sutures splay >3 mm in infant, sprung in older child; digital markings (also found in normal children), enlargement of the pituitary fossa, erosion of the clinoids.

Suprasellar calcification in craniopharyngioma.

CT is not as good as MRI at demonstrating posterior fossa abnormalities and spinal tumours or cysts.

Treatment

Surgery and irradiation according to site and malignancy of tumour. Chemotherapy pre-irradiation may improve results in under 3 year olds. Growth may be affected after pituitary irradiation, so requires pituitary function tests and follow up.

Prognosis

5-year disease free survival (and as a % of all childhood brain tumours in brackets): cerebral astrocytomas 25% (25%), cerebellar astrocytomas 95% (20%), medulloblastomas 50% (20%), brainstem tumours and ependymomas 20% (10% each), craniopharyngioma 80% (5%) with 10% postoperative mortality.

BENIGN INTRACRANIAL HYPERTENSION

Definition

Headache +/– diplopia, 6th nerve palsies, blurred vision, vomiting. Papilloedema and haemorrhages may be present. Follows recurrence of otitis media, steroid withdrawal, minor head injury.

Pathophysiology

Intra- and extracellular oedema, mechanism unknown.

Investigations

CT scan normal. LP diagnostic (>140 mm CSF), often therapeutic!

Treatment

LP. Dexamethasone is used if the intracranial pressure is elevated for prolonged periods of weeks or months, as vision is at risk.

Prognosis

Some children are left with minor deficits.

INTRACRANIAL BLEEDING

1   Trauma, accidental and non-accidental. Immediate danger of subdural and extradural haematomas. Chronic subdural collections may follow.
2   Spontaneous subarachnoid haemorrhage: rupture of arteriovenous malformation or aneurysm in 60%. Sudden onset, severe headache, meningism, apyrexial.

Prognosis

Mortality 20%, influenced by avoiding LP!

Further reading

Brett E M (1991) *Paediatric Neurology* 2nd edn. Edinburgh:Churchill Livingstone
Faerber E N (1986) Cranial computed tomography in infants and children. *Clinics in Developmental Medicine No 93*. Oxford: Blackwell
Fenichel G M (1988) *Clinical Pediatric Neurology. A Signs and Symptoms Approach.* Philadelphia:Saunders
Stephenson J B P and King M D (1989) *Handbook of Neurological Investigations in Children.* London: Wright
Weiner H L, Urion D K, Levitt L P (1988) *Pediatric Neurology for the House Officer.* 3rd edn. Baltimore:Williams and Wilkins

Index